This book is a basic guide for young adults (and newly diagnosed adults) with celiac disease (CD), also known as celiac sprue, nontropical sprue, gluten intolerance, gluten-sensitivity, and gluten-induced (or sensitive) enteropathy.

Due to the ever changing and evolving discoveries regarding celiac disease, this book serves as a reference only.

Elizabeth Atkinson

(2009)

*GLEE!*
An Easy Guide to
<u>Gl</u>uten-Fr<u>ee</u> Independence

by Elizabeth Atkinson

Copyright © 2009 by Elizabeth Atkinson

Cover Design Copyright © 2009 by Jeffrey A. Thompson

SmartList is a trademark of Clan Thompson LLC. All other names and trademarks contained in this publication are the property of their respective owners.

Published by Clan Thompson LLC

Clan Thompson LLC
42 Green St.
Bridgton, ME 04009

Printed in the United States of America

Online at: http://www. clanthompson.com

ISBN: 978-0-615-28165-0

*For my daughter, Brigitte*

*(aka: Malou)*

# FOREWORD

There is so much to worry about when you first leave home. Having safe food to eat shouldn't be one of them.

Like many parents with a teenager approaching adulthood, I've started to wonder, and worry, about whether or not I've given my son the skills to live on his own. On top of that, he has celiac disease and I also worry that he won't take proper care of himself when he ventures out on his own.

That's why, when Elizabeth Atkinson came to me with a book targeting young adults and the newly diagnosed, I jumped at the chance to publish it. There must be many parents of celiacs in my position, who would love a simple guide to hand to their kids as they head off to college or their first apartment. A guide that covered all the basics in an approachable way.

Well now they have one. Elizabeth has done an excellent job of taking such a large subject and covering it in an easy-to-read guide. It covers a bit of everything, from advice on getting gluten-free food at college, to safely sharing an apartment and the basics of preparing food. It also lists many resources to explore for further information.

There is enough to worry about when you first leave home. For those with celiac disease, this book takes care of one of the big ones.

Jeffrey A. Thompson

"The belly is the commanding
part of the body."

- Homer

# TABLE OF CONTENTS

*Getting Started*

# LEAVING THE NEST

We finally unraveled our daughter's tightly knotted digestive system at the end of her junior year in high school. Although her lifelong symptoms were on the moderate side, it suddenly became clear one day that her body did not tolerate gluten. As soon as we eliminated wheat, barley, and rye from her diet, our once semi-moody, rather-sleepy, always-crampy daughter blossomed into a very different person.

**Example**

Brigitte: "Do you need help with the dishes Mom?" (smiling)
Me: "Huh?" (passing out from shock)

I have never liked referring to Brigitte's condition as celiac disease (CD), because I do not feel she is "diseased" in any way. She is now healthy, happy, and filled with positive energy! (Well most of the time, unless you ask her younger brother.) Also, I have never fancied the term "gluten-free" because, frankly, it is not the most appetizing expression in the world. So in our house we refer to gluten-free food as "*Glee*" food.

**Example**

........................................................................

Brigitte: "Is this bagel *Glee*, Mom?"
Me: "No, the *Glee* bagels are in the *Glee* container."

Nowadays, Brigitte is getting ready to go off to college. The problem is she's still not altogether familiar with feeding herself *Glee* food. Eating is no longer as simple as throwing open the kitchen pantry after school and feasting on packaged, artificial, fabulous junk. In other words, I am now her personal (guilt-ridden) chef as I cook for her, bake for her, toast for her, chop for her, stock a cabinet just for her...you get the picture. And when dining out with her friends Brigitte still makes painful mistakes.

**Example**

---------------------------------------------

<u>Brigitte</u>: "I thought French fries were *Glee*, Mom." (grabbing her sore stomach)
<u>Me</u>: "Not when they share the same oil as breaded onion rings." (grabbing the hot water bottle and a cup of green tea)

As a result, I decided I better whip up a quick how-to-survive-without-thinking-about-it-too-much booklet for Brigitte before she stepped out into the big unknown world of totally pampered collegiate life. She has had no interest in reading the 300-page *Glee* books I ordered through our local bookstore or scanning one of the many immensely informative online *Glee* websites. Listen, she won't even slice her own orange.

**Example**

---------------------------------------------

<u>Brigitte</u>: "Will you slice an orange for me?"
<u>Me</u>: "You're in the National Honor

Society and you can't slice an orange?"

Brigitte: "Pleeeeeeease, Mom?"

Me: "Ugh."

So, for Brigitte and all those other daughters and sons living the *Glee* lifestyle as independent young adults (as well as anyone who has been newly diagnosed and totally overwhelmed)  tuck this book in your purse or backpack or glove compartment. When in doubt, pull it out and check it. Write in it, earmark it, highlight it—it's yours to personalize. I even left some blank pages at the end for you to add your own special notes or illustrations.

And may everyday be a *Glee*-ful day!

# WHY CAN'T SOME PEOPLE EAT GLUTEN?

"Gluten" is a term referring to the storage proteins found most commonly in wheat, rye, and barley. Gluten found in these grains gives a sticky or binding quality to foods.

Millions of people (particularly throughout the western world) are gluten-intolerant. Whenever they eat, drink, swallow (even lick) anything with gluten, their autoimmune systems react abnormally by kicking into gear and producing antibodies to fight the ingested gluten...basically rejecting the gluten. These fighting antibodies attack the small digestive system and actually damage it by destroying the tiny hairs or fingers called "villi". If the damage continues, the destroyed villi in the small intestine increasingly lose their ability to absorb certain nutrients from all food, possibly causing malnutrition.

This chronic condition, known as celiac disease (CD), never goes away. It is a genetic (hereditary) disorder, affecting as many as 1 in 133 Americans,* which *worsens without a gluten-free diet.* In fact, repeated (daily) gluten-induced attacks to the damaged intestine of someone with celiac disease will compromise the immune system and may allow other diseases to intrude.

The symptoms for celiac disease can begin to occur at any point in one's life from infancy up through old age. These symptoms vary enormously, but often include severe to moderate diarrhea and/or constipation and/or gas along with possible bloating and pain. Many people also have additional symptoms such as skin rashes (Dermatitis Herpetiformis), fatigue, joint/back pain, hair loss, low iron (anemia), inadequate growth/failure to thrive (in babies/children),

---

* "The prevalence of celiac disease in the United States has been estimated to be as high as 1 in 133 individuals. At the same time, only 1 in 4,700 individuals have been diagnosed with celiac disease. The average delay in diagnosis for a person with symptoms is 11 years. On average, a child will visit eight pediatricians before being diagnosed with celiac disease."
(Univ. of Chicago Medical Center: Celiac Disease Center www.uchospitals.edu/specialties/celiac/)

weight loss, irritability, infertility, and even depression. Some individuals have no symptoms at all, but are eventually diagnosed through other diseases, such as osteoporosis.

Since celiac disease is linked to other serious disorders, it is important to establish whether or not one has celiac disease. This can be done (with varying degrees of accuracy) by taking a blood test, a genetic test, or having a biopsy. First-degree relatives of an individual diagnosed with celiac disease should also be tested.

It is possible for individuals to have the symptoms of celiac disease, but not test positive for the condition. For reasons not fully understood, these individuals also benefit from a gluten-free (GF) diet.

**The Good News!**

___

While there is no cure for celiac disease, treatment does not require shots or pills. In fact, there is only one thing you must do (or not do!) to recover completely and to look and feel fantastic:

## DO NOT EAT GLUTEN FOUND IN
## WHEAT, BARLEY, RYE (and OATS)*

Unfortunately, avoiding gluten is easier said than done. Wheat and barley, in particular, are often hidden in foods where you wouldn't expect to find them. For example, wheat is sometimes used in soy sauce and barley is sometimes used in soy milks. In addition, many packaged and commercial foods rely on gluten as an ingredient in order to enhance the texture, taste, or quality of processed foods.

However, it is far easier to live gluten-free today than it was even five years ago!  Not only has mandatory allergy labeling begun to appear (see page 88), but today the general medical community is much more familiar with celiac disease. And since CD is possibly one of the largest health epidemics of our time, managing a gluten-free (GF) diet will only get easier.

* See page 10.

## The Big Three

**Wheat:** The most common "gluten offender," wheat is pervasive throughout our western diet in various forms. Baked items get their light, yet dense texture from wheat gluten. Other foods, such as condiments and gravies, achieve a creamy consistency with wheat gluten. Wheat thickens, stabilizes, and enhances so many foods we eat, it can be difficult to avoid.

**Barley:** Malt is commonly derived from barley, found in beer and malt vinegar, for example. Also, pearl barley is sometimes added to soups and stews. Beware of foods advertised as "wheat-less," as they sometimes contain barley.

**Rye:** The rye grain is found particularly in breads, crackers, and occasionally alcohol, such as rye beer. While rye is easier to avoid than wheat and barley, it is still found in mainstream cooking.

## What About Oats?

Oats do not have the same gluten proteins found in wheat, barley, and rye; however, there is a subset of people with CD who react to oats. Furthermore, commercial oats are often grown alongside fields of wheat and processed in the same facilities as wheat. Consequently, cross-contamination—which refers to the transfer of gluten from wheat, barley, or rye to another food that does not normally contain gluten—can occur. <u>Therefore, oats are generally safe to eat for those who tolerate them, but only if the label states that the oats were grown and processed by a gluten-free dedicated facility</u>.

*If you decide to include oats in your diet, let your doctor know so that you are regularly tested.*

## LET'S TALK

From chatting with my daughter and other young adults (and some older adults!) who are gluten-intolerant, one recurring complaint pops up over and over again:

> *You are sick of thinking about food, talking about food, eating food; and you definitely have little to no interest in cooking food.*

This is a maturity issue and will either subside substantially or disappear as you age into full, ripe adulthood. Promise. If not, marry or partner with a nutritionist or professional cook. Only kidding...<u>you will get used to *Glee* living and you will be fine</u>.

Of course, if you were raised in a culture where no one ate gluten, this would not be a problem. Since you do live in a wheat-eating, gluten-glutton world, you now need to shift your food perspective a bit. You have to pause and re-teach yourself what to eat. That's all.

Once you rebuild your knowledge of what you can eat, it will become second nature and you will not have to think about it. Of course, you will always have to ask questions when you dine outside your *Glee* household, but MANY people have food restrictions due to life-threatening allergies, religious observances, conditions, sensitivities, medications, eating disorders, and over-active gagging reflexes. You have a right to be upset, but eventually you will have to stop whining and get over it—it's just food. You will feel better, look better, and live a longer, healthier life!

# BASIC RULES

1   DO NOT STARVE—Do not let yourself get to the point where you are staaaaarving. This stresses your already sensitive stomach. Then you overeat and further upset that lovely digestive tract.

2   GRAZE—Learn to eat smaller amounts throughout the day. Keep snacks near you or accessible (e.g., purse, backpack). If you are served a large meal, eat half, then save the other half for later whenever possible.

3   MIX IT UP—Many *Glee* eaters repeat the same meals because they are reliable and easy. Add something new to your meal each time, like chopped pecans on your rice or sprinkle dried cranberries on your salad.

4   STOCK UP—Whenever possible, have a variety of staple *Glee* foods on hand, those items you can always count on to satisfy your appetite, such as *Glee* lentil soup, pasta, pretzels, bars, and crackers. Be sure to always keep a loaf of *Glee* bread in the freezer as well.

5    GET EXTRA FIBER—Eliminating wheat reduces your intake of fiber, which you need all the way down to your bowels. Make sure to eat plenty of whole grains (like brown rice and quinoa), fruits and vegetables.

6    DO NOT SHARE—Our parents may have taught us to share, but *Glee* eaters simply must avoid sharing items such as condiments and containers with their non-*Glee* eating friends and family. A ketchup bottle that comes in contact with a wheat hamburger bun is just as toxic to a *Glee* eater as taking a bite of the bun itself (see page 84).

7    VITAMINS—Consult with your doctor/nurse practitioner/nutritionist about vitamin and mineral supplements. People with CD are sometimes depleted of specific vitamins and minerals. Don't guess. Get expert advice. And make sure the vitamins and supplements are *Glee*. Call the company—they are happy to tell you. There should be a website or toll-free number listed on the label.

8    CHECK-UPS—At your yearly physical, you may want to have your blood tested to see if gluten is still present in your system. If so, consult with your physician to get at the source of the exposure. Rethink what you are eating (especially if you dine out or eat oats), and recheck medications as well as possible sources of cross-contamination (see page 84). And always use reputable Internet *Glee* sources to research foods/products.

9    NOT SURE?—Always check and double-check ingredients. But if you still aren't sure, don't eat it. Never risk ingesting gluten; it's not worth it. That includes *anything* that goes into your mouth, not exclusively food (see page 71).

10   EAT "REAL" FOOD—It is pretty easy to figure out which fresh, natural foods are gluten-free (GF). It is the processed, "convenience", packaged foods that make it difficult. So stick to fresh food most of the time.

11   ASK—Don't ever hesitate to stick up for yourself and ask. Ask the waiter to check the ingredients,

ask the chef at your college dining hall, ask your girlfriend's mother, etc. This may be the hardest part about eating *Glee*. And it's a pain, I know. But I promise you, it will get easier each time.

*A few ways to politely ASK:*

1   This all looks wonderful, Mrs. Eames, thank you. You may have heard I am allergic* to wheat and gluten, which is hidden in lots of foods like salad dressing. May I ask you what is in this dish?

2   I am anxious to try many things on your menu, but I need to ask the chef, which are gluten-free? Would you mind asking for me?

3   I am calling about your line of soups. I would like to purchase them but need to know which ones contain gluten. Thank you, I'll hold OR yes, please call me back!

It only takes a minute or two....

* CD is not an allergy, however, that is often the easiest way to describe it to others.

# ROOM AND BOARD

If you will be living and/or boarding at a small college or a huge university or an exclusive prep school or a 4-H camp or (fill in the blank)...

## Call Ahead and Meet and Talk with

1   The dining hall general manager (sometimes called the kitchen or cafeteria manager) and
2   The head chef of the dining hall/cafeteria and
3   The cafeteria office manager/assistant (who often does the shopping)

For the most part, they will have heard of celiac disease (CD). If not, they are well aware of food allergies and religious observances. In other words, it is their job to feed you.* If, for any reason, you sense tension or resistance, you should not attend that school or

---

\* Celiac disease is covered by the ADA, so register yourself at the Disability Office at your college/school/camp of choice to ensure *Glee* food is properly supplied.

camp unless you are prepared to take on your own meals. In our extensive East Coast college search, Brigitte and I found that every school cafeteria we visited was familiar with the *Glee* requirements and no one implied that it would be a problem or inconvenience in any way. In fact, some colleges even reserve a gluten-free corner with *Glee* breads and cereals.

The head chef at the college Brigitte will be attending in the fall asked us to sit down with him again at orientation to give him a list of her favorite meals, recipes, and snacks.

Brigitte will have her own *Glee* toaster in the cafeteria kitchen since heating elements are not allowed in the dorms. The chef has a designated *Glee* storage area in the cafeteria refrigerator and a separate cabinet shelf, and he will shop for Brigitte at the local health food store.

## Dormitory Appliances

---

Most dormitories allow a refrigerator as large as 4.6 cubic feet with a little freezer space. You should have the maximum size and keep it well stocked with healthy foods and snacks. It will also be necessary for you to bring a microwave to heat up quick meals. Many dormitories have a communal kitchen. If you opt to use a shared refrigerator and microwave, make sure you follow the appliance instructions on page 29.

## Breakfast

---

Many kids in college prefer to eat breakfast on the run or in their dorm room as they get ready for class. You should register for a 14-meal plan (2 meals/day each week) or less if you plan to *not* eat breakfast in the cafeteria. Instead, store GF breakfast items in your room.

## Lunch

---

Give the kitchen a list of meals you like for lunch, such as sandwiches (with gluten-free bread), soups, yogurt, etc. You may find you will make lunch yourself in the cafeteria, such as a *Glee* bagel with peanut butter. Again, lunch is often on the run between classes/activities, so remember to make sure the cafeteria has plenty for you to eat quickly. And give them ample notice when they are low on *Glee* foods.

## Dinner

---

When we asked the college chef if Brigitte will have to wait until after everyone else to get her dinner, the chef replied, "Absolutely not! Of course she will want to relax and eat at the same time as her friends." Eating in the dining hall, especially at dinnertime, is as much a social event as it is a time to refuel.

The chef offered good suggestions/tips for Brigitte to eat dinner comfortably:

1   Call an hour ahead from her dorm room before she eats to let the chef know what she would like and approximately when she will be arriving.

2   Give the chef recipes from home.

3   Choose one or two *Glee* dinners for the chef to cook in triple quantities on Sunday to store in the cafeteria fridge for the week. That way Brigitte can

arrive at any time, ask for a plate on the spot, or go in the kitchen and heat it up herself.

4   If nothing has been planned and Brigitte arrives unexpectedly for dinner (for example, after a late volleyball practice), she should let the chef know she is there and then head for the salad bar to join friends. He will heat up some lentil soup or chili on the spot and send it out to her table.

**NOTE:** Often, there are many assistant chefs in a kitchen and the head chef may not only be intimidating, but also very busy! Eventually you may find you click with one particular assistant chef. If that is the case, don't hesitate to talk with the kitchen manager and ask that you work and communicate with that one person.

# COMMUNICATION IS KEY

FYI...when I asked Brigitte how she felt about this friendly arrangement with the college chef, to my surprise she groaned and said how much she *hated* thinking about it and talking about it.

It is totally normal and understandable to feel upset about having CD. You have a million other things to worry about when starting out in a new living situation, particularly when school is involved. It is a royal pain to have to think about what you stuff in your mouth. Plus, you don't want to feel different from everyone else.

I reassured Brigitte that once she gets into the cafeteria routine, it will become second nature and her new friends will get over it as well. However, if there are kitchen problems, she will need to chat with the chef to let him know. If they still aren't resolved, then I will meet again with the staff to help smooth out any issues. Also, like any industry, there is a great deal of turn-over in the restaurant business, so you will likely have to deal with a new chef at some point.

I can't say it enough...communication is the key. Tell your parents/guardians, relatives and school counselor how you feel. And by all means, tell the chef. You (and/or your family) are paying a lot of money for your schooling or boarding experience.

REMEMBER: It is the kitchen's job to feed you correctly, comfortably AND deliciously! *And it's your job to thank them.*

# ELEVATOR SPEECH

As you may have already discovered, people constantly want to know what CD is or what gluten is or what your problem is. You may even find your friends challenging you, as if the condition is in your head. This is especially true for young adults who eat socially everyday in high school or college cafeterias where other teenagers are happy to pick at anything different.

It can be difficult to be patient, but think of it as a chance to educate others. Keep your answers short and simple, and then change the subject.

The following is an example of a GF "Elevator Speech" (i.e., prepared answer) to that never-ending question: "What's celiac disease?"

*"Celiac disease is a condition making me unable to digest gluten, which refers to the proteins found in wheat, barley, and rye. If I eat anything with gluten it makes me really sick for at least a day plus it damages my intestine every time I eat it . . . so did you watch the baseball game last night?"*

# BRING IT OR WASH IT

You have just arrived at your college dorm or your first shared apartment or your camp cabin as a counselor for the summer and you MUST get a few of the kitchen basics organized that first day.

## The Toaster

It is best that you not share a toaster with the wheat-eaters. BRING YOUR OWN PERSONAL TOASTER. Write clearly on the toaster in marker: "GLUTEN-FREE". However, if you must share, use a toaster oven (or the broiler rack in an oven) as the crumbs drop below. Always give the toaster oven metal grill a cleaning swipe. *Note:* Toaster bags are available to purchase online (www.toastitbags.com) if you must share.

## The Cutting Board

Again, it is best to have your own. In marker write: "GLUTEN-FREE". If you must share a cutting board, avoid wooden ones and wash thoroughly with hot water and soap before using.

## The Microwave

---

When sharing a microwave, make sure your item is on a plate or in some kind of container. Do not place your food directly on the microwave glass thingy that spins.

## The Pans & Utensils

---

Always best to have your own, but not as important as the toaster or cutting board! Before you use a shared pan or utensil, wash it first in warm water and dish soap.

## The Fridge

---

Do not store your leftovers in a container with your roommate's pizza or your *Glee* food will suffer cross-contamination. In other words, store your gluten-free food in your gluten-free containers. Again, write "GLUTEN-FREE" on the lids with a marker.

> **NOTE:** Always use your own sponge to clean, and wipe dry with either your own dishtowel or a disposable paper towel.

# HOG IT TO YOURSELF

---

Politely let people know that you have a food allergy\* and cannot share spreads and condiments. Remember to write "GLUTEN-FREE" on your containers, such as:

- Your butter or margarine
- Your cream cheese or sour cream
- Your jams
- Your condiments (mustard, mayo, ketchup, relish, etc)
- Your peanut butter
- Your salsa, dips
- Your sugar bowl

\* CD is not an allergy, but sometimes it is the easiest way to explain it.

# APARTMENT APPLIANCES

If you're cooking independently, the following appliances will make your life more delicious and nutritious!

## Slooooooow Cooker

A wonderful appliance and a must for the *Glee* eater, especially one who hates to cook. Slow cookers are affordable, available in different sizes, and usually come with nifty little recipe books full of easy stews and soups.

Before work or school, throw a bunch of yummy ingredients in the slow cooker, switch it on, and arrive home to a fabulous aroma...not to mention a nutritious meal that usually lasts a few days!

## Bread Machine

There is nothing like fresh hot bread, no matter the grain! Most (for Brigitte, "all") of the pre-packaged gluten-free sliced breads are pretty awful. And the freshly baked *Glee* breads can cost as much as $10 per loaf! There are many types of bread machines on the market, so look around. If you don't want to make bread from scratch, start with gluten-free bread mixes (such as Gluten-Free Pantry Favorite Sandwich Bread Mix) which adapt to bread machines.

## Blender

One of the best ways to get in your daily dose of dairy and fruit is to make a smoothie. We use organic frozen fruit (in place of ice chips), good French vanilla yogurt, fresh chopped fruit, and a little pure bottled fruit juice (like peach or mango). You can also use your blender to make wonderful cold vegetable juices and soups, like Gazpacho.

# THE GROCERY STORE

Shopping for *Glee* food is no longer the huge issue it used to be. Once traditionally offered only by health food stores, gluten-free options are now available at almost all mainstream supermarkets.

Generally, *Glee* food is divided into three sections at the grocery store:

1   Gluten-free shelf items
2   Frozen gluten-free items
3   Naturally gluten-free foods (such as fruit, vegetables, meat, dairy, etc) , often referred to as the "perimeter foods" since they are usually found along the outside aisles of a grocery store.

Some markets (such as Whole Foods, Trader Joes or Wegmans) will even give you a published list of all gluten-free products found throughout their store. Others (like Whole Foods) prepare and bake their own line of *Glee* items!  Many times *Glee* food is shelved on or near the organic food aisles. Never hesitate to ask at the customer service desk for help at any supermarket to speed up your search.

When Brigitte and I inquired about GF products at a local, independent grocery store, the manager enthusiastically offered to give us a GF tour as well as personally type up a list of GF items!

By the way, eating a gluten-free diet is perfectly fine* for everyone, not just people with CD! If one or two members of a household need to go *Glee*, the whole household should. Ultimately, it creates less stress when shopping and prevents the kitchen from becoming contaminated by wheat (yuck) and other gluten sources. (Just remember to get extra fiber.)

* A gluten-free diet has recently become "trendy" and confused with the popularity of "fat-free" or "sugar-free" or "carb-free" diets. There are no proven benefits or drawbacks for a normally healthy person to eat gluten-free other than to make a kitchen safer for someone with CD.

*The Lists*

# ASK AGAIN AND AGAIN AND AGAIN AND...

The following section contains three lists of general guidelines about:

1   what you <u>can eat</u>
2   what you should <u>avoid or question</u>, and
3   what you <u>cannot eat</u>

I do not know all the ice cream brands that are gluten-free or which bolognas contain gluten. Furthermore, manufacturers change their ingredients from time to time.

Find a few brands you like and stick with them. If you have questions about the ingredients, look up the toll-free phone number on the container; then call and ASK. Why? *Because the toll-free number is there for consumers to ask questions.*

I know it is bothersome and annoying and makes you want to scream, but once you find out that, *yes! your favorite ice cream and bologna are Glee,* you can jot it down in the back of this book and run out and buy some!

The problem occurs when "the expert on the phone" does not know or isn't sure. They may be able to tell you that their product does not contain wheat, but they aren't positive about the gluten. Or they may not know the source of an ingredient in their product, such as a spice mix. Or they may inform you that they make other products with gluten, so there is cross-contamination. These are the times when you have to make your own decision about the product.

Luckily for you, there is practically a gluten-free alternative for everything these days. Brigitte told me she missed graham crackers the most–and a good old fashioned S'more. I found *Glee* graham crackers on the Gluten-Free Mall (www.glutenfreemall.com). Then I researched which marshmallows are GF (like Jet Puff) and I already knew plain Hershey bars are *Glee*. The only problem was getting the fire started, but we prevailed.

# YES—YOU CAN EAT—*GLEE* LIST!

**YES!** *(the following PURE grains, flours, and their pastas)*

| | |
|---|---|
| Amaranth | Arrowroot |
| Besan | Buckwheat (not a wheat plant) |
| Cassava | Fava bean |
| Flax | Gram flour (not graham) |
| Lentil flour | Millet |
| Montina | Nut flour |
| Polenta | Potato flour |
| Psyllium | Quinoa |
| Rice bran | Rice flour |
| Sorghum | Soya flour |
| Tapioca flour | Teff |
| Wild rice | Yam flour |

**YES!**

✓ Bacon and eggs (except soufflés or egg casseroles made with wheat flour)
✓ Baking soda, cream of tartar, baking yeast (check baking powder)

- ✓ Beans, lentils and legumes (includes most baked beans like B&M, Bush's)
- ✓ Boar's Head deli meats
- ✓ Cellophane noodles, pure rice noodles, pure rice wrappers
- ✓ Cheese (except some brands of processed cheese, cottage cheese, cream cheese, Stilton, Gorgonzola, blue, and Roquefort)
- ✓ Cheetos (most varieties—check website)
- ✓ Chocolate—plain (many, like Nestles and Hershey's)
- ✓ Coffee and tea (question flavorings, bottled, and instants)
- ✓ Corn tortillas and corn taco shells (pure corn flour)
- ✓ Cornmeal, corn flour, corn starch—pure corn anything!
- ✓ Dairy products (for the most part, and if you are not lactose intolerant)
- ✓ Distilled liquor, wine (properly distilled liquor and wine to which no gluten-containing ingredients were added following distillation—see page 74)

- ✓ Doritos tortilla chips (most, like Cool Ranch, Spicy Nacho and Taco Flavored; *Nacho Cheese are not Glee,* so check to make sure formulations have not changed)
- ✓ Fats such as butter and oils (check margarine/spread ingredients)
- ✓ Fish, canned (like Bumble Bee and Chicken of the Sea tuna, sardines, anchovies, clams, salmon, oysters)
- ✓ Fresh meat and fresh fish
- ✓ Fruit and vegetables
- ✓ Ice cream, plain (most, except those with obvious added cookie/brownie globs. Also, some chips/nuts may have been dipped in wheat.)
- ✓ Sherbet, sorbet, frozen yogurt
- ✓ Jams and jellies/preserves (most, but check)
- ✓ Ketchup (most, like Heinz)
- ✓ Marshmallow Fluff
- ✓ Mashed potatoes (without flour to thicken), fried potatoes/hash browns, baked potatoes, french fries (pure oil), any potatoes
- ✓ Mayonnaise (most, like Hellmann's)

- ✓ Mustard (most, but be cautious of mustards due to malt vinegar)
- ✓ Nutella
- ✓ Nuts, including nut butters (peanut butter, almond butter, etc.) and pure nut flours

> **WARNING:** packaged nuts may be coated to prevent sticking, check label

- ✓ Old El Paso seasonings
- ✓ Ore-Ida Tater Tots
- ✓ Pickles, olives
- ✓ Popcorn in almost all forms, except some of the flavored ones
- ✓ Potato chips, plain (not all potato chip snacks, like sticks and stacked chips)
- ✓ Rice Chex by General Mills (a commercial brand cereal!)
- ✓ Salsas—homemade and some jarred (Ortega, Newman's Own, Green Mountain Gringo)
- ✓ Soda (most commercial brand sodas—check gourmet specialty sodas)

- ✓ Soups, clear (most, like Progresso and Healthy Valley, but check)
- ✓ Spam
- ✓ Sugar, brown sugar, honey, real maple syrup, powdered sugar
- ✓ Tacos/tortillas (made from pure corn, no wheat)
- ✓ Tomato paste and most tomato sauces
- ✓ Velveeta cheese (but not all processed cheese products)
- ✓ Vinegar (except malt)

# AVOID OR QUESTION—*GLEE* LIST

*This list pertains mostly to store-bought, pre-packaged, and restaurant items since you know what is in your homemade food!*

## AVOID or QUESTION

? Baking powder (usually okay, but check)

? Barbecue sauce, cocktail sauce (lots of additives, so check)

? Buckwheat (despite it's name, pure buckwheat is not wheat but related to rhubarb—however, wheat is often added to many buckwheat products, so must be labeled GF)

? Candy corn (a few GF brands available, such as Goelitz)

? Canned liquids, vegetable broth, gravy cubes, bouillon (some are okay)

? Caramel color (almost always made with corn, but manufacturers are allowed to use barley so it should be checked)

- ? Chili, canned (homemade is fine, as are some canned varieties like Hormel)
- ? Condiments (many are okay and some are already labeled "gluten-free", like Annie's)
- ? Cotton candy
- ? Creamy salad dressings (study ingredients on all salad dressings if not labeled GF)
- ? Egg rolls (wrappers usually made with wheat)
- ? Emulsifiers, enzymes
- ? Energy bars
- ? Energy drinks, "bottled" coffees and herbal teas
- ? Fat replacements (found in some low-fat foods to give a "full-fat" flavor—some may contain gluten, such as Nutrim)
- ? Flavored chips, flavored nuts, flavored popcorns, flavored milk, flavored anything (unless labeled "gluten-free")
- ? Generic soda and juice drinks (juice that is not 100% pure)
- ? Hamburger and meat patties (may have fillers at restaurants)
- ? Herbal supplements

- ? Highly processed cheeses and dairy products
- ? Hot dogs which have a variety of fillers (Wrangler, Boars Head beef franks are okay)
- ? Ice cream bars and shapes (some are okay, like Dove Bars)
- ? Low-fat food (generally GF with the exception of some fat replacements)
- ? Marshmallows (many are okay, like Jet Puff, but check)
- ? Modified food starch (usually corn starch is used in food, which is fine, but question all starch in medications)
- ? Prepared meats/deli meats (may have marinades or herbal rubs, be pre-stuffed or pre-basted—but Spam is *Glee*)
- ? Rice cakes and some rice crackers (check ingredients)
- ? Rice mixes (boxed) may contain "fillers"
- ? Rice syrup (may include barley)
- ? Sauces, marinades, thickened or pasty liquids
- ? Soups (creamy, chunky—check!)
- ? Spice blends and commercial seasonings

? Tuna and chicken salad at restaurants (some add bread or fillers to stretch the quantity)

? Veggie burgers (often contain wheat)

? Vitamins/mineral supplements (may contain "fillers" with gluten)

# GENERAL—DO NOT EAT—*GLEE* LIST

## NO: WHEAT ~ BARLEY ~ RYE (OATS*)

**NO:** *wheat in all forms*

---

| | | |
|---|---|---|
| Bran | Bulgur | Cake flour |
| Couscous | Durum | Einkorn |
| Emmer | Farina | Frumento |
| Fu | Graham | Kamut |
| Matzo | Orzo | Seitan |
| Semolina | Spelt | Tabbouleh |
| Triticale | | |

**NO:** *ingredients using the word "wheat"*

---

Wheat germ oil (also called triticum vulgare), wheat nuts, wheat protein, wheat starch, wheat grass, etc.

\* It is considered acceptable by most experts to eat oats if they are tolerated, but only if they are grown and processed by dedicated gluten-free companies with appropriate labeling. However, if you include oats in your diet, let your doctor know so you can be regularly tested.

## NO

- ⊘ Food that has been *breaded, floured, stuffed,* served in a *sauce* made with wheat or wheat derivatives (including *cheese sauces*), *marinated* in a sauce that contains gluten, such as *soy sauces* or *teriyaki sauces*...unless it is prepared with *Glee* alternatives.
- ⊘ Bakery items: breads, muffins, pastries, pancakes, rolls, cookies, cakes, pies, bars (unless labeled "gluten-free")
- ⊘ Beer or non-alcoholic beer (unless it is labeled "gluten-free" and you are 21 or older)
- ⊘ Bisque or chowder or gravy or roux (unless it is made with *Glee* flour)
- ⊘ Breakfast cereals (unless labeled "gluten-free"; usually found in the natural food aisles)
- ⊘ Brewers (or nutritional) yeast (regular baking yeast is fine)
- ⊘ Communion wafers (generally, you may request GF wafers by calling ahead)
- ⊘ Crackers, biscuits, pretzels, ice cream cones (unless GF)

- ⊘ Deep fried food: onion rings, chicken nuggets, and commercial french fries due to cross contamination (unless french fries are specifically cooked in a dedicated fryer and have not been rolled in additives)
- ⊘ Egg soufflés, egg dishes, egg casseroles (unless you know what has been added)
- ⊘ Flavored commercial sauces, dips, cheeses—just skip them or make them yourself!
- ⊘ Imitation crab/fish meats (watch for use in sushi and salad bars)
- ⊘ Imitation nuts and coated nuts
- ⊘ Licorice (unless labeled "gluten free") or jelly-type candies (unless you have contacted the company)
- ⊘ Malt, malt syrup, malt extract, malt flavoring, malted milk, malt vinegar, malt anything (unless specified that it is derived from corn—most malt derived from barley)

  EXCEPTION: Malt dextrin (or maltodextrin) is a sugar and is generally gluten-free, unless labeled that it is derived from wheat.

- ⊘ Miso (red type contains barley, but yellow should be fine)
- ⊘ Ovaltine or Postum
- ⊘ Pizza (unless labeled "gluten-free")
- ⊘ Pastas including lasagna, ravioli, etc. (unless labeled "gluten-free")
- ⊘ Potato casseroles or "dishes" (unless you know what has been added)
- ⊘ Rice Dream (currently contains barley) and some soy milks
- ⊘ Sprouts from barley or barley grass (no barley anytime)
- ⊘ Stilton, blue cheese, Gorgonzola or Roquefort (traditionally, these cheeses are made with bread, but some commercial types are not)
- ⊘ Stuffing (unless prepared with GF bread) or stuffed foods and meats
- ⊘ Udon noodles (unless made from corn) or soba noodles (unless made from pure buckwheat)

# WHAT-ARE-THEY-ANYWAY?
## *GLEE* LIST

---

**YES:** *it is okay to ingest*

---

- ✓ Agar and algin
- ✓ Annatto color
- ✓ Aspartame (artificial sweetener)
- ✓ Benzoic acid
- ✓ BHA/BHT
- ✓ Calciums (chloride, lactate, phosphate, etc.)
- ✓ Carob
- ✓ Carrageenan
- ✓ Citric acid
- ✓ Fructose
- ✓ Fumeric acid
- ✓ Glycerin
- ✓ Hydrolyzed meat protein
- ✓ Isomalt (artificial sweetener)
- ✓ Lactid acid
- ✓ Lactose

- ✓ Maltodextrin or malt dextrin (a "malt" exception, unless labeled made from wheat)
- ✓ Mono/diglycerides (unless noted on the label that they contain a wheat carrier)
- ✓ Monosodium glutamate or MSG
- ✓ Monostearates
- ✓ Niacin
- ✓ Nitrates/nitrites
- ✓ Oleic acid
- ✓ Palmitate
- ✓ Pectin, pectinese
- ✓ Pepsin
- ✓ Potassium iodide
- ✓ Propylene glycol monostearate
- ✓ Protease
- ✓ Rennet
- ✓ Riboflavin
- ✓ Sodium (ascorbate, ascorbic acid, benzoate, citrate, nitrate, stearoyl lactylate)
- ✓ Stearic acid
- ✓ Sucrose

- ✓ Tri-calcium phosphate
- ✓ Vanillin

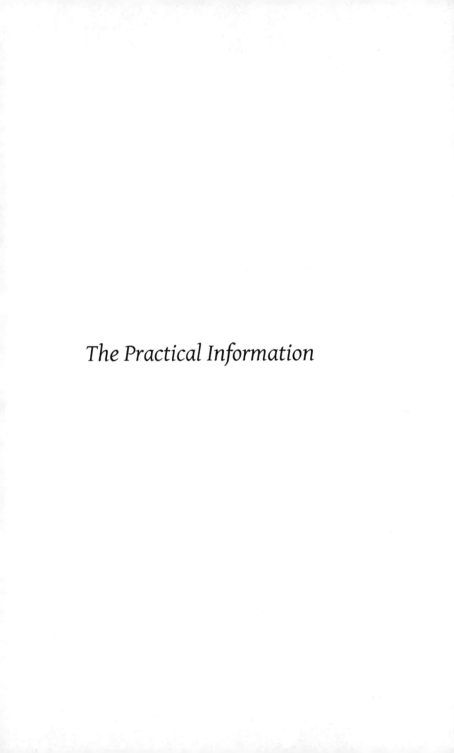

*The Practical Information*

# PIZZA, CHIPS & SODA

## Pizza

Obviously, the crust of mainstream pizza is very gluten-ful, made from wheat flour. However, the rest of pizza ingredients (tomato sauce, fresh parmesan and good mozzarella cheese, topped with oregano and basil) are naturally *Glee!* So you can make your own scrumptious pizza with *Glee* crusts sold in many grocery stores. Also many companies (such as, **By George**, **Amy's**, **Glutino**) sell a good *Glee* pizza in the frozen GF section. And **Chebe** makes a wonderful pizza crust.

More and more independent pizzerias and restaurants (like *The Boynton Restaurant* in Worcester, MA and *Pizza Luce* in St. Paul. MN) offer delicious *Glee* pizza. Ask around—it's more common than you think!

## Chips

Plain potato chips and corn chips are *Glee!* However, some of the flavored ones are not. Also, many chips are not made on a dedicated gluten-free line, so cross-contamination may occur. You need to do the research and decide. Here is a starter list:

*Glee Chips*

-------------------------------------------------------------------

- ✓ Plain potato chips
- ✓ Frito Corn Chips
- ✓ Lays Stax
- ✓ Doritos Cool Ranch
- ✓ Cheetos
- ✓ Plain tortilla chips

*Non-Glee Chips*

-------------------------------------------------------------------

- ⊘ Barbecue potato chips (often not GF)
- ⊘ Barbeque corn chips (often not GF)
- ⊘ Pringles (a few varieties are now GF)
- ⊘ Doritos Nacho Cheese
- ⊘ Some "baked" chips
- ⊘ Some "flavored" chips

## Soda

Generally speaking, soda is gluten-free. There is some concern about caramel coloring and whether or not it is derived from barley. Rarely are caramel colorings derived from barley due to the high cost. However, there may be gourmet or "boutique" sodas with unusual ingredients, especially some root beers. To be on the safe side, you need to check the ingredients of your favorite sodas, but here is a starter list:

*Glee Sodas*

- ✓ Coke/Diet Coke
- ✓ Mountain Dew
- ✓ Barq's Root Beer
- ✓ Pepsi Cola
- ✓ Sprite/Diet Sprite
- ✓ Mug Root Beer
- ✓ Orangina
- ✓ Yoo-Hoo

- ✓ Dr. Pepper
- ✓ Schweppes Ginger Ale
- ✓ Slice
- ✓ Fresca
- ✓ Canada Dry Ginger Ale

## Other *Glee* Beverages

---

- ✓ Gatorade
- ✓ PowerAde
- ✓ Propel
- ✓ Nesquik
- ✓ Capri Sun
- ✓ Red Bull Energy Drinks
- ✓ Swiss Miss Milk Chocolate Cocoa
- ✓ Starbucks Frappucino Beverages
- ✓ Hershey's Chocolate Syrup & Cocoa
- ✓ Nestles Coffee-mate

# CANDY, GUMS & MINTS

Yes, you may still eat many disgustingly delicious, packaged candy bars and confections.

HOWEVER, this is an ever-changing list. Plus, a candy bar made for the US market may have different ingredients in Canada or other parts of the world. <u>And many manufacturers adjust their ingredients each year</u>.* To top it off, most of these candies are not produced in gluten-free kitchens.

Pick out the few candy bars you like and stick to them if you must indulge occasionally—nothing wrong with that! Call the company to make sure they are currently gluten-free. Recheck ingredients with the company every year.

Call the toll-free phone number listed on the label or website to double-check ingredients. The list below does not include all gluten-free candy, gums and mints. Many of these items are not produced in guaranteed

---

* **Disclaimer:** Formulations can change and information can become out of date, so check product labels prior to using.

wheat-free environments, so there may be cross-contamination.

> **NOTE:** To be on the safe side, <u>do not purchase</u> any of these candies in *special shapes,* such as a peanut butter cup "egg", without calling the manufacturer first. Sometimes, manipulated candy products need fillers to hold them together and the fillers may contain gluten.

## Suggested *Glee* Candies*

---

- ✓ Andes Mints (all)
- ✓ Baby Ruth Chocolate Bar
- ✓ Butterfinger Chocolate Bar (not including Butterfinger Crisp or Stixx)
- ✓ Cella's Dark Chocolate Covered Cherries
- ✓ Cella's Milk Chocolate Covered Cherries

* Clan Thompson Gluten-Free Food "SmartList 2009" (CANDY): www.clanthompson.com

- ✓ Charleston Chew (all)
- ✓ Charms Blow Pops
- ✓ Dagoba Dark Chocolate bars (all)
- ✓ Dots (Mason-Tropical–Wild Berry)
- ✓ Dove Chocolates (all–except Milk and Dark Chocolate Covered Almonds)
- ✓ Dum Dum Pops
- ✓ Fluffy Stuff Cotton Candy (made by Tootsie Roll)
- ✓ Gimbal's Black & White Licorice Mix
- ✓ Gimbal's Organic Fruit Bears
- ✓ Gimbal's Sugar-Free Black Licorice Scottie Dogs
- ✓ Green & Black's Hazelnut and Currant Bar
- ✓ Green & Black's Maya Gold Bar
- ✓ Green & Black's White Chocolate Bar
- ✓ Haribo's Gold-Bear Gummi Bear (original)
- ✓ Jelly Belly Jelly Beans
- ✓ Junior Mints
- ✓ Let's Do Organic Classic Gummi Bears
- ✓ Life Savers Hard Candy
- ✓ M & M's (plain & peanut)
- ✓ Milky Way Midnight Bar (NOT the original)
- ✓ Nestle Bit-O-Honey

- ✓ Nestle Goobers
- ✓ Nestle Milk Chocolate
- ✓ Nestle Milk Chocolate Nest Eggs
- ✓ Nestle Nips (regular and sugar-free)
- ✓ Nestle Raisinets
- ✓ Nestle Sno-Caps
- ✓ Nestle Spree Candy Canes
- ✓ Nestle Treasures (including Treasures Bars)
- ✓ Nestle Turtles (milk chocolate–dark chocolate–sugar-free)
- ✓ Nestle Valentine Milk Chocolate Hearts
- ✓ Newman's Own Organics Chocolate Bars–Milk Chocolate
- ✓ Peeps Chicks (blue, lavender, white, pink)
- ✓ Peeps Cocoa Bunnies
- ✓ Peeps Ghosts
- ✓ Peeps Pumpkins
- ✓ Reed's Ginger Chews
- ✓ See's Candies Licorice Medallions
- ✓ Smarties
- ✓ Snicker's Almond Bar

- ✓ Snicker's Candy Bar
- ✓ Spangler Candy Canes
- ✓ Spangler Circus Peanuts
- ✓ Starburst Fruit Chews
- ✓ Starburst Jelly Beans
- ✓ Sugar Babies
- ✓ Sugar Daddies
- ✓ Teuscher Chocolates (all except French nougat and Florentine)
- ✓ Three Musketeers Bar
- ✓ Tootsie Fruit Rolls
- ✓ Tootsie Pops
- ✓ Tootsie Rolls
- ✓ Wonka Gobstoppers (chewy and original)
- ✓ Wonka Laffy Taffy (Rope and FruiTart chews)
- ✓ Wonka Lik-M-Aid Fun Dip
- ✓ Wonka Mix-Ups
- ✓ Wonka Nerds Gum Balls
- ✓ Wonka Pixy Stix
- ✓ Wonka Shockers
- ✓ Wonka SweeTARTS

- ✓ Wonka SweeTARTS Lollipops
- ✓ Wrigley's Crème Savers Hard Candies

## Suggested *Glee* Gum and Mints

---

- ✓ Adams Black Jack Gum
- ✓ Altoids Mints
- ✓ Beemans Gum
- ✓ BreathSavers Mints
- ✓ Dentyne Gum (peppermint, spearmint, arctic chill, spicy cinnamon)
- ✓ Dentyne Fire Mints
- ✓ Dentyne Ice Mints
- ✓ Hubba Bubba Bubble Gum
- ✓ Trident Gum (original, spearmint, bubblegum, cinnamon)
- ✓ Wrigley's Big Red Gum
- ✓ Wrigley's Freedent Gum
- ✓ Wrigley's Juicy Fruit Gum
- ✓ Wrigley's Orbit Gum
- ✓ Wrigley's Spearmint Gum

## NEVER EAT!

---

- ⊘ Twizzlers (some brands of licorice, like Candy Tree, are GF)
- ⊘ Anything with "Malt" (like Whoppers)
- ⊘ Jelly-type candies (unless you contact the company)

*Candy with cookie base or ingredients:*

- ⊘ 100 Grand Bar
- ⊘ Kit Kat
- ⊘ Krackle
- ⊘ Milky Way (original)
- ⊘ Nestle Crunch
- ⊘ Reese's Stix
- ⊘ Take 5
- ⊘ Twix
- ⊘ Whatchamacallit

# MY MEDS

Many over-the-counter and prescription medications use cornstarch as a filler, but sometimes wheat or other gluten-containing grains are used in both name-brand and generic meds, so they always need to be checked. Call the manufacturer of over-the-counter meds! When ordering a prescription, automatically ask the pharmacist if it is gluten-free. This includes <u>allergy medicines</u>, <u>birth control pills</u>, and <u>antibiotics</u>. There is a good chance they will not know, but it is their job to find out for you.

**Generic**

It's important to know, too, that just because your generic medicine is gluten-free one time, it may not be the next time. Generic meds are made by different manufacturers and your pharmacy may change their suppliers. Make sure you check your generic meds every time you fill your prescription. Your prescription bottle should list the name of the generic manufacturer right on the bottle. If not, ask your pharmacist.

> **NOTE:** Check meds before you get your prescription filled or while you're still in the drugstore. If you wait until you get home, and the ingredients turn out *not* to be gluten-free, you won't be able to return the prescription.

The following is a list of some generally accepted over-the-counter *Glee* medications. As always, this list is not guaranteed. You should double-check with the manufacturer to make sure the ingredients have not changed. Also, call the manufacturer of your vitamins and supplements to ensure they are *Glee*.

Call the toll-free phone number listed on the label or website to confirm ingredients. Remember: Formulations can change and information can become out of date, so check product labels prior to using.

The list below does not include all gluten-free, over-the-counter medicines. Many of these items are not produced in guaranteed wheat-free environments, so there may be cross-contamination.

**Suggested *Glee* Over-the-Counter Medicines***

---

✓ Actifed Cold & Allergy Caplets

✓ Advil

✓ Afrin

✓ Alavert

✓ Alluna

✓ Anbesol

✓ Benadryl Elixir, Allergy & Cold Tablets, and Inhaler

✓ Blistex Lip Balm

✓ Bufferin tablets

✓ Bugs Bunny Chewable Vitamins

✓ Chapstick Lip Balm (regular)

✓ Claritin

✓ Dayquil

* Sources: www.glutenfreedrugs.com; and Clan Thompson Drug SmartList 2009–www.clanthompson.com

- ✓ Excedrin Extra Strength
- ✓ Fibercon and Fiberlax
- ✓ Gas-X chewable tablets (not the soft gels)
- ✓ Imodium and A-D Caplets
- ✓ Lactaid Original Strength Caplets
- ✓ Metamucil (not wafers)
- ✓ Motrin
- ✓ Neosporin Original
- ✓ Nicoderm CQ
- ✓ Nicorette (mint)
- ✓ NyQuil
- ✓ Pepto Bismal Caplets
- ✓ Preparation H
- ✓ Primatene Mist & tablets
- ✓ Robitussin
- ✓ Rolaids
- ✓ Sominex
- ✓ Sudafed
- ✓ Sunkist Multivitamin Complete
- ✓ Tamiflu
- ✓ Tavist
- ✓ Theraflu Cough and Cold

- ✓ Triaminic Chest and Congestion
- ✓ Tums (all except Smoothies)
- ✓ Tylenol
- ✓ Vaseline
- ✓ Vicks (Adult 44, cough drops, DayQuil, Inhaler, Ny-Quil, Sinex Spray)

# DO NOT LICK, SUCK, CHEW, KISS...

Believe it or not, there are other items and individual mouths you should think twice about before bringing to your lips. They either contain gluten or may remotely contain gluten, so avoid licking, sucking, chewing, or kissing them.... Many are gross anyway, so just keep them out of your mouth. You could accidentally ingest trace amounts.

## Check ingredients of:

| | |
|---|---|
| Chalk | Cosmetics |
| Envelopes | Glues |
| Hairsprays | Hand lotions |
| Household cleaners | Lip balm |
| Lipstick* | Play-doh |
| Shampoos, gels | Soaps |
| Stickers, stamps | |

* most common offender

## About Kissing...

- If you kiss someone wearing lipstick or cosmetics (which may contain gluten) OR
- If you kiss someone who has just sipped a beer OR
- If you kiss someone who has just eaten a wheat-a-ful turkey sandwich OR
- If you kiss the hand of someone with hand lotion (which may contain gluten) OR
- If you kiss a dog that has rolled in gluten-filled garbage...

...you may experience cross-contamination.
Wash up afterward and brush your teeth, rinsing thoroughly.

### *Glee* Toothpaste

The following toothpaste manufacturers make toothpaste which is gluten-free. Check the labels and/or double-check their websites to make sure they have not changed their ingredients.

Arm & Hammer

Pepsodent

Crest (Proctor & Gamble)

Tom's of Maine

**NOTE:** Most <u>mouthwash brands</u> and <u>whitening strips</u> are gluten-free, but not necessarily all. Check the ingredients or call the manufacturer.

## The Dentist

Let your dentist (as well as all of your doctors and specialists) know that you have CD and insist s/he checks the ingredients of those substances entering your mouth.

---

In America, you can vote, get married, fight in wars, live on your own, have babies, drive a truck, and buy cigarettes by the time you turn 18. But, as you know, it is against the law to drink alcohol until you are 21 years old. There are various pros and cons for and against this law.

Just remember, liquor impairs your judgment... potentially causing you to vote for Homer Simpson, father a child with someone you met at a bar, or start a nasty nicotine habit. However, for those of you 21 and older who enjoy an occasional imbibing, most alcohol is *Glee* because it is distilled. <u>Beer, malt liquor, and some liquor with added flavorings are not gluten-free.</u>

**Wine\***

---

Wine is naturally gluten-free. This includes champagne, sherry, vermouth, sake, and sparkling wines.

\* Some wine makers age their products in barrels sealed with a flour paste. It is unclear if this process causes cross-contamination.

However, double-check wine coolers as some contain "malt" liquor (which is a no-no).

## Vodka, Rum, Whiskey* and Gin

---

All of these distilled liquors are gluten-free. When adding mixers, check the labels. Tonic water and club soda are *Glee*.

## *Glee* Beer

---

*Many gluten-free beers are now available.* Once, only overflowing with non-distilled malted barley, beer used to be totally forbidden. But now there are many gluten-free labels on the market. In fact, our local liquor store has a gluten-free banner hanging above one section of beer. Most of the *Glee* beers are made from gluten-free sorghum. They differ quite a bit in taste, so be sure to sample the different brands (which are labeled "gluten-free").

* Some whiskey makers age their products in barrels sealed with a flour paste. It is unclear if this process causes cross-contamination.

## Liqueurs

---

Brandy, Schnapps, Cognac, Kahlua are all *Glee,* as are many others. But do the research first.

## Margaritas? Pina Coladas?

---

The liquor (tequila, rum) is gluten-free, but, again, the added syrups/mixes are not always *Glee.* The safest way to enjoy a mixed drink is to use fresh ingredients and make it yourself.

## DO NOT DRINK...

---

⊘ **"Malt" Beverages** *(generally contain barley):*
Do not drink any liquor that contains the word "malt" on the label or in the ingredients, unless it says it is specifically made from corn. Aside from beer, this also includes the flavored beverages, wine coolers, and those that begin with the word "Hard" (Hard Ice Tea, Hard Lemonade, Hard Cider, etc).

- ⃠  **Beer:** Unless labeled "gluten-free."  This goes for non-alcoholic beer as well.
- ⃠  **Flavored alcoholic drinks or mixers:** Until you find out if they are gluten-free.

# RECHARGE YOUR BATTERIES

While the guidelines below are advisable for everyone to follow, it is particularly important for the *Glee* individual to live well in order to regain energy, promote a healthy immune system, and stabilize those bowels.

1   SLEEP—Get 8+ hours of sleep every night and try to stick to a regular sleep schedule, even on the weekends.

2   WATER—Generally speaking, drink half your weight in ounces of water on a daily basis. If you weigh 140 pounds, drink 70 ounces of water/day (about six 12-ounce glasses of water/day). Obviously, if you're hot or playing sports, drink more.

3   GENTLE EXERCISE—Walk 30 consecutive minutes every day, preferably outdoors. Stretch.

4   EAT—Dark green vegetables (like spinach!) every day and tomatoes often.

5   LAUGH—Do whatever it takes to laugh each day—even if it requires sitting in a park with your dog and making fun of people.

6   SING–Do it in the shower, do it in the car, but learn to sing out loud no matter how bad you sound. (It may take care of #5.)

7   MEDITATE–Nothing fancy. Just sit in a comfortable, unlit, quiet space. Attempt to empty your mind by concentrating on or counting each breath. Inhale and exhale evenly and slowly for about 5 minutes each day.

8   AVOID CAFFEINE–Replace coffee with herbal tea whenever possible, don't consume caffeine after lunch, and rarely (if ever) drink soda.

I often hear *Glee* individuals (won't name any names) complain:

"I HATE MY STOMACH!"

These individuals do not want you (or anyone) to touch their stomachs, look at their stomachs, or talk about their stomachs. In fact, a person with CD will often ignore their own stomach like a giant boil between their chest and thighs.

For years, his/her agitated gut has been bloated, burning, tender, distended, crampy, bubbly and blubby, aching, squeezing, shredded...well, you know what I mean.

The good news is their digestive tract (and yours) is on the mend. Even though it may take a year or more before that belly feels healed, it's time to start forgiving it now and welcoming it back to the rest of your body.

"How?" you ask...

1   Give your stomach a loving pat every morning.

2   Gently exercise your stomach with a few sit-ups or deep breathing exercises.

3   Cuddle up with a hot-water bottle.

4   Learn to Belly Dance or Disco or Hula (originally a man's dance). If you don't want to take a class, buy a DVD or a book and shake it!

5   Get a cool henna tattoo on your stomach.

6   Above all, apologize to your stomach for all those terrible months/years of mistrust, betrayal, and agony. And then promise to cherish your digestive tract for as long as you both may live.

Like a snowflake or a silky cobweb or a butterfly wing, a glattack (i.e., gluten attack) is unique to each person.

Unlike a snowflake, or a silky cobweb, or a butterfly wing, a glattack is usually a hideously unpleasant experience.

However, you will make mistakes and you will have glattacks. While they are miserable, a glattack is not the end of the world. And eventually you will learn to avoid them.

**NOTE:** While some people know exactly what a glattack feels like, others cannot easily discern between a glattack and some other type of stomach ache (such as, an allergy or even a plain old stomach bug). If you are unsure of your glattack, first review your diet/symptoms to see if there could be another reason why you are not feeling well.

Write down what you ate the hour(s) or so before the glattack. Keep the list on the fridge or somewhere easily accessible. The glattack may be the result of cross-contamination (see next page) or it may be that the person who informed you is incorrect ("yes, *all* our medications are gluten-free, sir...").

# CROSS CONTAMINATION

## Possible Hidden Sources of Gluten Contamination

- French fries deep-fried in common oil used for breaded foods (ASK!)
- French fries rolled in mysterious coating (Why do they taste funny?)
- Vegetables steamed in used water, such as pasta water (It's possible!)
- Burgers/chicken grilled where buns have been grilled (double check)
- Old wooden cutting boards, wooden utensils, and serving items (toss)
- Dirty silverware trays (You have to clean those?)
- Condiments shared with wheat-eaters (Get your own jar!)
- Somebody is using your toaster (Geez, I hate that!)
- Toothpaste brand (Check everything that goes in your mouth)
- Your girlfriend's peach flavored lip balm (see page 71)

# A WORD ABOUT EMERGENCIES

Some experts and doctors differ on emergency situations, so it is up to you to decide if you should wear a medic alert bracelet or necklace.

Our nurse practitioner thinks it is unnecessary (and possibly dangerous) to wear one as celiac disease does not present an immediate life-threatening reaction. If an emergency worker hesitates or becomes confused about what to do, life-saving measures might be withheld.

However, our nurse practitioner does recommend carrying a note in your wallet which identifies your celiac disease and explains you cannot ingest gluten. And make sure your doctor confirms on the front of your chart that you have CD and that you require a gluten-free diet.

# DID YOU KNOW?

- Gluten cannot be absorbed through the skin. However, you need to wash your hands regularly so traces of gluten do not land in your mouth.

- It is now estimated that possibly 1 in 133 people in the USA may have celiac disease/gluten sensitivity; and as many as 90% are not yet diagnosed, as most have "silent" symptoms.

- Italy, the pasta capital, has one of the highest incidences of celiac disease in the world. In fact, children are commonly screened for CD in Italy upon entering first grade.

- People with many other ailments, such as diabetes, thyroid disease, autism, mental illness, colon afflictions may significantly improve their health on a gluten-free diet.

- Breast milk is naturally gluten-free.

- The adjective, *glutinous*, does not describe something with gluten. It refers to anything sticky like molasses.

- Even celebrities and professional athletes have celiac disease (search it on the Internet).

- Confirmed celiac disease precludes you from serving in the US military.

- Dog food is full of gluten. For heaven's sake, don't eat it and after serving Fido, wash your hands. (PS: There are gluten-free dog foods available.)

- You may be able (with detailed receipts) to deduct gluten-free expenses, including food, from your taxes. For more information, contact: Internal Revenue Service www.irs.gov (800) 829-1040.

# US LAW ON LABELING

The FDA passed an allergy labeling law that said, as of January 1, 2006, all food containing wheat must list the ingredient on the label (along with milk, eggs, peanuts, tree nuts, fish, shellfish, and soy). Even though wheat is the main enemy of a gluten-free diet and by law must now be disclosed on labels, you still need to look out for barley, rye, and oats. They are not required to be listed on allergy warnings.

**Standard VOLUNTARY Gluten-Free labeling\* should *begin to* appear throughout the US!**

The FDA had planned to write the US definition of "gluten-free" by the end of 2008 in order to begin labeling food products, but the deadline came and went. *However*, once the definition is finalized, gluten-free

---

\* For more information, refer to the *US Food and Drug Administration:* Questions and Answers on the Gluten-Free Labeling Proposed Rule (www.cfsan.fda.gov/~dms/gluqa.html)

labeling will be voluntary and not mandatory. Consequently, many smaller companies who manufacture gluten-free foods and products will choose not to use the designation due to additional costs. Therefore, you will still need to read labels and check ingredients.

*Dining Out and Travel*

# RESTAURANT TIPS

1   Call ahead to see if you need a reservation. Then inform the host that you (or someone in your party) require gluten-free food. If the host immediately recognizes your condition and assures you that they have gluten-free choices, book a table. If they have no idea what you're talking about, skip it.

2   Upon arrival, identify yourself to the host and then your waiter.

3   Eat a healthy snack before you go out in case your meal is inedible.

4   It is always safer to order "naked" food. A meal consisting of a plain meat, a plain starch like rice or potato, and steamed vegetables* is the safer way to go.

5   Remind your server that pans/grill must be clean and free of gluten.

* Make sure vegetables are steamed in pure water, not leftover pasta water.

6   Bring your own dessert like a piece of dark chocolate or a gluten-free cookie to have with a cup of tea or decaf coffee after dinner.

7   Eat at restaurants with gluten-free menus. It's more common than you think! (See following list of national restaurant chains)

8   Refer to websites at the back of this book, which list restaurants with gluten-free menus/options by zip code or state.

9   Check out www.opentable.com—a reservation service which allows for comments on your dietary needs.

10  Try to develop a relationship with a particular restaurant that will become familiar with your gluten-free needs. Some may even allow you to bring in your own GF soy sauce or breads for the kitchen to use.

# RESTAURANT CHAINS

The following national restaurants have dedicated *Glee* menus or information online and/or on location:

**Biaggi's:** www.biaggis.com

**Bonefish Grill:** www.bonefishgrill.com

**Boston Market:** www.bostonmarket.com

**Carrabba's Italian Grill:** www.carrabbas.com

**Cheeseburger in Paradise:**
www.cheeseburgerinparadise.com

**Chili's:** www.chilis.com

**Fleming's Steakhouse:** www.flemingssteakhouse.com

**Legal Sea Foods:** www.legalseafoods.com

**Mitchell's Fish Market:**
www.mitchellsfishmarket.com

**On the Border:** www.ontheborder.com

**Outback Steakhouse:** www.outback.com

**P.F. Changs:** www.pfchangs.com

**Romano's Macaroni Grill:** www.macaronigrill.com

**Taco Del Mar:** www.tacodelmar.com

**Ted's Montana Grill:** www.tedsmontanagrill.com

**Uno Chicago Grill:** www.unos.com

**Wildfire:** www.wildfirerestaurant.com

# FAST FOOD TIPS

One of the hardest parts of having CD is being spontaneous. What do you do when a friend (or group) suggests stopping at a pizza place or a fast food joint?

1   Don't panic or be afraid to go along with the friend/group.

2   Possible items you can order:
- *French fries* (ask if there is a dedicated fryer AND if there is a coating on the fries)
- *Soda*
- *Plain salad* (made fresh)
- *Plain ice cream*
- *Burger* (fresh with no bun on a cleaned or dedicated grill)
- *Grilled chicken sandwich* (fresh with no bun on a cleaned or dedicated grill)
- *Baked potato* (plain with butter/sour cream/real bacon)
- *Bag of plain potato or corn chips*

3   If you order a plain salad, request it be made with no croutons and a clear dressing on the side (such as Italian or oil & vinegar).

4   Ask if the hamburgers are pure meat or if there are fillers (see page 100). Ask if the grilled chicken was ever in marinade or has additives (skip if it had either). A burger/grilled chicken must be made fresh, that is, *not removed from a bun.*

5   <u>If you don't want to ask any questions</u> or make a request (such as no croutons), be safe and just buy a soda and a bag of plain chips.

6   <u>If you don't mind asking questions</u>, ask if they have a GF menu (see list of fast food restaurants on the next page) or anything GF on their menu. (Brigitte had a friend in high school who always insisted on asking for her). If they don't have a GF menu/item, then make the inquiries suggested above.

# FAST FOOD CHAINS

The following fast food restaurants list *Glee* information on their websites.* When stopping at one of the fast food restaurants listed below, feel free to ask for their gluten-free menu. If the person at the register has no idea what you mean, inform them that they have a gluten-free menu online and ask that they please check it. They may need to ask a manager to help, but don't hesitate to ask. They want you to buy their food!

**Wendy's:** www.wendys.com

**Burger King:** www.burgerking.com

**Kentucky Fried Chicken:** www.kfc.com

**Pizza Hut:** www.pizzahut.com

**Taco Bell:** www.tacobell.com

**Arby's:** www.arbys.com

**Chikfila:** www.chikfila.com

**Dairy Queen:** www.dairyqueen.com

* When "wheat" and "gluten" appear under "Allergens" in an online menu refer to the "gluten" column (celiac disease is not an allergy, however that is the way in which the restaurant and food industries commonly refer to the condition).

**WARNING:** Remember—most fast food restaurants (and the majority of restaurants) deep-fry food in <u>shared oil</u>. That means those tasty French fries are probably skinny dipping with wheat-encrusted chicken fingers. And don't assume a plain burger without a bun is fine. ASK! Breadcrumbs or fillers may be added (to stretch the meat); grilled chicken (in sandwiches) may have been dipped in a mystery sauce before cooking, so ASK.

# ETHNIC RESTAURANTS

Generally speaking, Indian, Thai, and Mexican restaurants should have many gluten-free options if the food is freshly and authentically prepared. This is also true of some Near East, Middle East, Spanish Tapas, and North African menus. While many Asian restaurants have gluten-free foods, most use soy sauce in the kitchen. So even if soy sauce is not in the dish, cross-contamination may occur.

If you plan on visiting a truly ethnic restaurant it is a good idea to go online and print out a Celiac Dining Card explaining gluten-intolerance in the language of choice:

## www.celiactravel.com
*(click on: "Free Gluten-Free Restaurant Cards")*

Hand the card to the waiter and ask if you are able to eat any of their dishes. Again, if they seem confused I would not eat at that restaurant. If they are confident that they understand your condition, you should be fine.

**NOTE:** Many Italian restaurants seem to have gluten-free menus or options these days. This may be due to the fact that Italy has one of the highest celiac disease rates in the world.

# GO AHEAD AND TRY IT!

The following is a list of foods you may or may not have heard of which can be terrifically *Glee* (when prepared authentically and not thickened with flour, fried in shared oil, or made with gluten sources, such as some broths). Most are quick, nutritious and easy to eat. Just because they sound weird doesn't mean they taste weird. So go ahead and give them a try!

Many of these are available at ethnic restaurants (as well as major grocery stores and/or health food shops):

✓ Bean Vermicelli—Asian cellophane noodles (or glass noodles) made from mung beans.

✓ Béarnaise Sauce—A tarragon sauce served with beef; includes eggs, butter (similar to Hollandaise Sauce).

✓ Chicken Masala—Popular Indian dish containing chicken marinated in yogurt, cooked with incredible spices.

- ✓ Dolma—Greek in origin, grape leaves typically stuffed with savory rice, ground lamb, pine nuts and fabulous herbs and spices.
- ✓ Falafel—A Middle Eastern treat of spicy deep-fried ground chick-pea balls served with yogurt or tahini dip. (Often served in pita bread, so order falafel only and check oil.)
- ✓ Fruits—Papaya, tamarind, jujube, breadfruit, persimmon and guava.
- ✓ Hominy Grits—A hot cereal made from plain ground corn, usually eaten at breakfast in the southern states. (Make sure no wheat has been added.)
- ✓ Kulfi—Delicious Indian ice cream made with cardamom and nuts.
- ✓ Paella—Spanish dish with a base of rice, tomato and saffron. (Check broth.)
- ✓ Papadam—Large, peppery Indian cracker made from lentil or chickpea flour. (Check oil.)
- ✓ Ratatouille—An aromatic Mediterranean vegetable stew, delicious over rice. (Check to see if thickened with flour.)

- ✓ Remoulade–A French sauce made with mayonnaise.
- ✓ Risotto–Creamy Italian rice dish. (Check broth.)
- ✓ Sun Butter–Like peanut butter, but made from sunflower seeds; also try almond and cashew butters.
- ✓ Tahini–Another tasty butter made from ground sesame seeds.
- ✓ Tempeh–Patty packed with protein made from cooked soybeans.
- ✓ Veggies–Bok choy, kale, exotic mushrooms, leeks, jicama, spaghetti squash.
- ✓ Venison or Buffalo–Trendy meats, low in fat, high in protein.
- ✓ Wakame–Thin seaweed used in salads and Asian soups. (Check additives.)

# HEY SWEET TOOTH

There are many gluten-free desserts already available... *if prepared authentically*. Don't forget to double-check at restaurants and ask if anything non-*Glee* has been added, such as thickeners or stabilizers or flavor enhancers. Also, check to see if the baking pan has been floured.

### *Glee* Desserts

| | |
|---|---|
| Torte | Custard |
| Compote | Sorbet/Glacée |
| Chocolate Mousse | Jello (gelatin) |
| Fudge/Penuche | Crème Brule |
| Peanut Brittle | Rice Pudding |
| Praline | Tapioca |
| Coconut Ball (Thai) | Macaroons |
| Meringues | Toffee |
| Ice Cream (plain) | Frozen Yogurt (plain) |

## *Glee* Toppings

---

Chocolate or strawberry sauce (homemade ingredients), coconut (fresh), M&M's, nuts (make sure they aren't rolled in flour to prevent sticking), whipped cream (homemade ingredients).

> **WARNING:** Some marshmallows and marshmallow sauces are not gluten-free, so check ingredients.

# TRAVELING ABROAD*

It goes without saying, the free restaurant cards (see page 101) are crucial to the traveling *Glee* individual. Many countries, particularly throughout Europe and the UK, have very informative websites. Do your research before you travel and try to contact the Celiac Foundation in the country to which you are traveling.

For example, search "Ireland Celiac" and www.coeliac.ie† will pop up. When Brigitte and I traveled to Ireland, this fantastic organization immediately e-mailed a list to us including all the gluten-free restaurants, bed & breakfast accommodations, and grocery store information for the entire country! In addition, they gave me their contact numbers to call them while

---

* **IMPORTANT NOTE:** While US Celiac Association standards currently define gluten-free food as maintaining zero traces of gluten sources, European standards are not quite as rigid. The discrepancy remains controversial throughout the international celiac community. For up-to-date information, please refer to: www.csaceliacs.org and search "definition of gluten free."

† In many English-speaking countries Celiac is spelled, "Coeliac," but pronounced the same.

we were there. Needless to say, I popped a money order donation in the mail and a heartfelt thank you note.

If you can't find your destination country after searching online, log onto www.clanthompson.com and click on "Resources", then "Contacts & Links" and scroll down to "Celiac Associations Around the World." If you still can't find your country, e-mail Clan Thompson. They will do their best to help you!

- Request a gluten-free meal on your flight. These days, very few airlines offer them. Even so, ask in order to educate.

- Carry enough *Glee* SNACKS/FOOD to last a minimum of twenty-four hours at the airports and on flights. You're in survival mode!

- Opt to RENT an apartment or a condo or a suite with a kitchen when traveling. It is best if you have the choice to do your own basic cooking.

- Look for GLUTEN-FREE TOUR GROUPS. There are many! Or think about taking a CRUISE—all the major cruise lines claim to accommodate the *Glee* diner if you contact them 3–4 weeks ahead of departure.

- Consider visiting those COUNTRIES with the HIGHEST INCIDENCE of celiac disease (and awareness), such as Canada, Italy, Ireland, Australia, Sweden, Finland, Norway, Denmark, Argentina, Austria, Israel. It makes traveling a lot easier.

- TELL EVERYONE: If you are traveling abroad with your college or a new job, let those in charge know that you must stick to a gluten-free diet.

- Bring 1 cup of BROWN RICE: We always travel with a container of brown rice. We immediately make it upon arrival and stick the pot of rice in the refrigerator, as anything (veggies, meat, cheese, etc.) can be added later. If you don't have a measuring cup, the container serves as one. The amount of water is a bit more than double the rice; bring to a boil, then simmer for 45 minutes until all water is absorbed.

- Drink SMOOTHIES! This is a great and simple way to get your daily fruit, vitamins, fiber and calcium (from the yogurt) when you're abroad. Ingredients are usually listed on the menu.

- Find the closest HEALTH FOOD STORE: They not only carry gluten-free items, but the employees can usually make suggestions for gluten-free restaurants, bakeries, etc.

- STOP IN restaurants when you're out shopping or touring during the day and ask if they are familiar with CD (show them the card).
- DON'T OVERDO IT! Don't plan an overly ambitious trip until you have the hang of it. And do as much research as possible before you leave. By all means, travel! But realize it may take some getting used to your special *Glee* limitations.

*Food Solutions*

## SIMPLE *GLEE* COMBOS

Whether you're dining at the cafeteria, eating at a friend's house, travelling on a class trip, or munching somewhere other than your cozy, gluten-free home, here are some quick and tasty meal ideas.

You can either assemble the following ingredients from a cafeteria/buffet line or order the ingredients separately at a restaurant. However, you must ASK about the ingredients to ensure they are *Glee*.

These are also quick meals I assemble for Brigitte on the go. Many of the ingredients may be prepared ahead of time and kept for several days in the fridge to mix up on a moment's notice.

Along with a salad or serving of fruit, any of the *Glee* combos below provide a quick and hearty meal!

- Rice, salmon, cooked broccoli (sprinkle with lemon)
- Mashed potatoes, sliced beef, sautéed mushrooms
- Brown rice, bacon pieces, chopped tomato (sprinkle with fresh parmesan cheese)

- Yams, dried cranberries, diced pork (add chopped pecans)
- Diced chicken or flaked tuna (plain) mixed with mayonnaise and chopped celery (eat with pure corn tortilla chips)
- Rice, chick peas, green peas (with butter or marg)
- Whipped potatoes combined with cooked hamburger, corn niblets (good with Heinz ketchup which is *Glee*)
- Lentil or bean soup, brown rice, sliced GF chicken sausage
- Baked potato, diced ham, cooked red peppers (with pure sour cream)
- Two eggs and 1 TBS cream cheese scrambled in 1 tsp. olive oil with handful of fresh spinach (and chopped tomatoes)
- Cellophane noodles (prepared) mixed with 1 TBS olive oil, cooked canned clams w/juice (lemon & pepper)
- Rice, cooked asparagus, feta cheese
- Chili! Fresh, pasta-free, clear soups! (made on-site, not packaged, ASK for ingredients)

- Rice noodles, any sautéed veggies, baked tofu (NO SOY SAUCE on or cooked with food unless GF soy sauce)
- Real corn tortilla or taco, black beans, fresh salsa (fresh cheese)
- Hash browns, omelet with green peppers
- Wild rice, trout (grilled), steamed cauliflower (add almond slivers)
- Grilled/broiled steak (check for marinade), corn on the cob, sautéed vegetables

# *LA SALADE* BAR

While salad bars may seem harmless, be wary of artificial items (e.g., imitation seafood, bacon bits) and creamy salad dressings or anything floating or coated in marinade. In addition, make sure your waiter doesn't pick out croutons from a prepared salad and serve it.

Try these quick combinations and mix up your own salad dressing (see page 120 for on-the-spot recipes!) Even bottled GF salad dressings can be hard on the sensitive *Glee* stomach.

- Spinach, dried cranberries, feta or goat cheese, chopped pecans (sweet dressing)
- Add to cooled rice: artichoke hearts, peppers, cocktail shrimp, scallions (tangy dressing)
- Fresh broccoli, sprouts (not barley sprouts), shredded cheddar, real bacon bits (creamy sweet dressing)
- Lettuce, apple pieces, chopped celery and walnuts (sweet dressing)

- Chick peas, cold green beans, red pepper, red onions (tangy dressing)

# ON-THE-SPOT SALAD DRESSINGS

---

**Estimate measurements on the spot**

---

1 level soup spoon =

about the size of a tablespoon (TBS)

1 level regular spoon =

about the size of a teaspoon (tsp)

*Mix up in a clean cup, taste, adjust, and pour!*

**Cold Dressing (sweet)**

---

- $1/_2$ TBS vinegar (red or white wine vinegar)
- 2 TBS oil (a light oil, like safflower, is best)
- $1/_4$ tsp mustard (Grey Poupon & French's are GF)
- 1 tsp maple syrup (OR honey OR sugar)
- (Optional: Add $1/_2$ TBS GF mayonnaise, like Hellman's, to make it creamy.)

## Cold Dressing (tangy)

---

- $1/2$ TBS vinegar (red/white wine or cider vinegar)
- 2 TBS olive oil
- $1/4$ tsp mustard (Grey Poupon & French's are GF)
- dash of herbs (i.e., basil, oregano, thyme, etc.) salt/pepper and/or garlic


**HOT Dressing:** *good on spinach salads, microwave cup of dressing 20 seconds and pour*

---

- 1 tsp oil
- 1 TBS cider vinegar
- 1 TBS honey
- $1/4$ tsp lemon juice

# ON-THE-SPOT DIPS

## Great for fries, hamburger

- 1 tsp mayo (Hellman's is GF)
- 1 tsp ketchup (Heinz is GF)

## Yummy with pork, chicken

- 1 TBS mustard (Grey Poupon & French's are GF)
- 1 tsp honey

## Nice with fish

- 1 tsp mayo (Hellman's is GF)
- 1 tsp chopped sweet pickles (most pickles are considered GF as they are made with distilled vinegar, however check all ingredients on pickles and relishes)

# PARTY DIPS

## Mild Guacamole

- a ripe avocado, mashed
- $^1/_2$ small tomato, diced
- 1 tsp lime juice
- 1 TBS fresh (or $^1/_2$ tsp dry) cilantro
- (Optional: Add a little chopped onion, garlic, chilies to spice up.)

## Egg Salad Spread

- Boil (gently) 3 eggs 7–8 minutes, cool, peel
- Mash 2–3 TBS mayo into egg (Hellman's is GF)
- Sprinkle with paprika or pepper or curry

## Light Veggie Dip

- 1 cup plain yogurt
- 2–3 TBS fresh dill weed (minced) or 2 tsp dried dill

- 1 small cucumber (peel and slice vertically in quarter lengths, then core out seeds, chop finely)

## Fishy Dip:

---

- 1 small can of salmon
- 2 oz. cream cheese
- 2 oz. sour cream

## Chocolate Dip: for Glee pretzels, cookies, strawberries

---

- $1/4$ cup chocolate chips (Nestles is GF)
- 1 tsp water

*Microwave 30 seconds, beat until creamy.*

## Peanut Butter Dip: *for apples and bananas*

---

- $1/4$ cup smooth peanut butter
- $1/6$ cup honey
- $1/4$ tsp cinnamon

**Frosting Dip:** *for GF cookies and/or cakes*

---

- $^1/_4$ cup butter or margarine (soft)
- 1 cup powdered sugar (sift into butter)
- 1 TBS milk (or strong coffee)
- (Optional: Include 2–4 TBS unsweetened powdered cocoa in powdered sugar.)

## Chip Dip

---

- Lipton Onion Dry Soup Mix (yes, it's *Glee*)
- 1 pt sour cream

**Syrup Dip:** *for GF waffles, pancakes, biscuits*

---

- 1 cup frozen blueberries
- 1 cup water
- $^1/_2$ cup brown sugar

*Cook on stove until hot.*

# READY-MADE *GLEE* DIPS

Spread on *Glee* crackers, use as a dip, or add as a condiment to any dish!

- ✓ Baba Ganoush
- ✓ Fresh Salsa
- ✓ Hummus
- ✓ Marshmallow Fluff
- ✓ Nutella
- ✓ Pesto
- ✓ Tahini

*Very* Basic Cooking

# HOME SWEET *GLEE* HOME

Whether you want to admit it or not, it's best to eat homemade meals—nutritionally as well as financially. While that's true for everyone, it is particularly true for the *Glee* eater...*so that you are in control of the ingredients.* Dining out should be an occasional treat.

I usually have a pot of cooked brown rice and/or a bowl of mashed potatoes and/or a container of prepared GF pasta in the fridge as a foundation for many quick meals. Frozen *Glee* breads are also good to have on hand. To any healthy carbs you can quickly add a bit of protein, a cooked vegetable, and a salad.

The following chapters include <u>basic instructions for food preparation</u>. They are not highly seasoned recipes, so experiment with additional spices, herbs and stuff from the fridge—along with the easy marinades I've included for meats (see page 156).

Once you understand the basics, venture out and buy a *Glee* cookbook!

# THE FILLING STUFF! (CARBS)

Carbohydrates make up about 45%–65%* of your daily intake and give you energy. While low-carb diets may be trendy, most experts agree that a generous amount of "complex" healthy carbs (whole grains, fruits, vegetables) are an essential part of a balanced diet.

## Rice

This incredible food sustains much of the world. However, it is nutritionally inferior when it is white or polished, which means it has been fully milled with the germ and bran removed. EAT WHOLE GRAIN RICE, which includes brown rice, wild rice, basmati brown rice and naturally colored (purple, red, or black) rice. Now you can even purchase par-cooked brown/wild rice with dried beans or lentils—delicious! Whenever possible buy *organic* whole grain rice.

* USDA: National Agricultural Library. "Dietary Reference Intakes: Macronutrients." Food and Nutrition Information Center (2008).

> **WARNING:** Before buying <u>rice mixes</u>, check ingredients as gluten may be added.

*To Prepare Rice*

Follow directions on the box. Cool before transferring to refrigerator. Keeps several days in fridge. Reheat single portions in microwave.

## Pasta

I have to admit, most of the *Glee* pastas we have tried are pretty weird. There are several varieties and you will just have to experiment until you find the type which appeals to your personal taste buds. Brigitte prefers the <u>rice-based pastas</u>, but there are also <u>soy</u>, <u>corn</u>, <u>quinoa</u>, and <u>combination pastas</u>.

Pasta is very versatile and keeps a few days in your fridge. To prevent it from sticking in clumps, toss the pasta in a bit of olive oil before it cools, then transfer it to a covered container and store in the fridge until you are ready to use it.

<u>Asian rice noodles</u> are delicious, light and easy to cook. They are terrific in clear soups or stews. To a plate of rice noodles, add stir-fried or steamed vegetables, almonds, peanuts, tofu, pork, scrambled egg, chicken, seafood, whatever! And since you are cooking at home, toss on some of that *Glee* Soy Sauce!

> **WARNING:** Some imported rice noodles contain small amounts of wheat. Check ingredients.

*To Prepare Pasta*

Again, follow directions on the box/bag. (We have found that the rice pastas/noodles cook quickly and can become mushy, while the other varieties may need to be overcooked as they tend to be chewy.)

## Potatoes

Yams/sweet potatoes are generally more nutritious than the white variety. White potatoes spike blood sugar, but they also provide potassium and other nutrients. Besides they're filling and delicious. So eat moderately and go light on the butter and gravy.

The skin of an organic potato is nutritious (like apples, carrots, etc.) and provides fiber, but can be hard on your delicate *Glee* stomach. I always recommend peeling, but it is up to you.

> **NOTE:** You can also cook parsnips or turnips along with potatoes for added nutrition.

*To Prepare Boiled Potatoes*

- Peel potatoes and rinse in cold water (so they don't turn brown).
- Cut into large, bite-size pieces.
- Drop into almost-boiling water and bring to a boil (use enough boiling water to cover the potatoes by 3").
- Boil (gently) 4–5 minutes for **par-boiled (firm) potatoes** or 7–8 minutes for **soft potatoes** (test by jabbing a potato with a fork).
- Drain in colander.

- Place desired amount in bowl, toss with a little butter or olive oil and eat, or use plain boiled potatoes in the recipes that follow. Extra potatoes should cool before transferring to the fridge. They last 3–4 days in the fridge.

*To Prepare Roast Potatoes*

-------------------------------------------------------------------

- Preheat oven to 375°F.
- Melt 1 TBS butter/marg in microwave, add 1 TBS olive oil and stir.
- Place 3 cups of par-boiled (firm) potatoes in a pan, cut if large.
- Pour butter/oil mixture over potatoes and toss thoroughly.
- Add salt and pepper (and herbs, such as rosemary/thyme or garlic).
- Bake about 30–45 minutes, depending on desired toasty-ness. Turn a couple times while roasting.

*To Prepare Baked Potatoes*

-------------------------------------------------------------------

- Preheat oven to 425°F.

- Wash potato skin well, pat dry.
- Pierce with fork several times.
- Bake for 1 hour (less for sweet potato/yams which also tend to drip, so place cookie sheet on lower rack).

*To Prepare Whipped Potatoes*

- Place 4 cups hot, soft boiled potatoes in bowl.
- Add $1/2$ cup milk (or soy milk, plain yogurt or goat's milk), 3 TBS butter/marg, salt, pepper.
- Whip with electric beater until smooth.
- (Optional: Instead of butter/marg add 4 TBS cream cheese. Also, add in a crushed garlic clove for great flavor.)
- ("Mashed" potatoes are typically made with less liquid and are mashed by hand.)

*To Prepare Fried Potatoes*

- Heat large frying pan to MEDIUM heat.
- Add 2 TBS Oil (or butter/marg) in pan (may add chopped onion, garlic).

- Toss in 3 cups of firm potatoes (chopped, diced or grated).
- Turn with spatula occasionally until potatoes are browned to your liking.

## Corn

---

Corn, right off the cob or frozen is delicious and filling. Avoid eating canned corn or creamed corn unless you know what has been added.

Ground corn is used in many ways from polenta to corn tortillas. As long as the item is cooked with pure corn flour, it is fine. And don't forget fresh, plain popcorn is a healthy snack, full of fiber.

---

**WARNING:** Commercial cornbread is off limits as it is made with wheat. Bakery items using corn must be labeled GF as corn flour is almost never used alone in mainstream baking. However home-made GF cornbread is easy to make!

---

## To Prepare Corn-on-the-Cob

......................................................................

- Fill a large pot with 3" water and bring to a boil.
- Husk the corn (break in half if too big for pot).
- Place in boiling water.
- Cover and steam for 5–7 minutes, turning once or twice.

## To Prepare Frozen Corn

......................................................................

Frozen corn is boiled–follow directions on package. Check ingredients of any frozen vegetables that include sauces/butters/creams.

## Bread

Like pasta, you will have to experiment with all the bread varieties. Many of the tastier breads are tasty to kids because they are made from white rice. They are not particularly nutritious, but fine on occasion and make better sandwiches. And most (if not all) *Glee* breads taste much better toasted.

We have yet to discover a delicious pre-made sliced bread; however there are some rice-based rolls that are tasty if well-toasted. Brigitte uses these rolls for sandwiches and as hamburger buns. She also likes a particular *Glee* sesame bagel and English muffin. Many people love Chebe bread and some breads are also nut based, so be adventurous!

> **NOTE:** Consider investing in a bread machine and begin with ready-made gluten-free bread mixes. Hot, fresh bread is always tasty!

### Pancakes/Waffles

There are countless *Glee* pancake mixes available, almost all delicious. Check to see they are made from brown rice rather than white. Add anything to the batter, such as blueberries, strawberries, apple bits, diced banana, chopped nuts, ground flax seed, or GF chocolate chips*. Don't forget to grease the pan before

* Many commercial chocolate chips are gluten-free, but always read over the ingredients.

spooning in the batter and make smaller ("silver dollar") pancakes. *Glee* varieties are not quite as firm as those gluten-filled ones, so the pancakes can be difficult to flip.

We always have a box of *Glee* waffles in the freezer. They last for weeks and make a quick, filling snack.

> **NOTE:** <u>Real maple syrup</u> is naturally GF. Check ingredients of artificial syrups.

### Instant/Quick Sources of Carbohydrates

If you don't have time to prepare a meal, the following foods provide an instant or quick source of carbohydrates:

- ✓ Canned beans
- ✓ Frozen corn
- ✓ Cold *Glee* cereal in milk
- ✓ Hot oatmeal (if you tolerate oats)
- ✓ Banana/apple
- ✓ Lentil GF soup

- ✓ Instant mashed potatoes w/o additives (Bob's Red Mill or Barbara's)
- ✓ Canned beets
- ✓ Popcorn (plain)
- ✓ Whole grain *Glee* breads
- ✓ Cream of Rice
- ✓ Rice cake and rice crackers (GF)
- ✓ Hummus

## Tasty Grain/Flour Alternatives

There are many delicious grains and flours to eat other than rice and corn. The grains all cook pretty much like rice and they last for days in the fridge. Try substituting one of these other flours in recipes that call for rice flour.

NOTE: Since many of these grains/flours may be processed in plants which also process wheat, purchase those labeled "gluten-free".

- ✓ AMARANTH (tasty nutritious seed, cooks like rice)
- ✓ ARROWROOT FLOUR (West Indian Marantha Arundinacea root)
- ✓ BESAN (chickpea flour)
- ✓ BUCKWHEAT (related to rhubarb, but make sure wheat has not been added)
- ✓ CASSAVA FLOUR (starch substitute)
- ✓ FAVA BEAN (whole or ground into a flour)
- ✓ FLAXSEED (seeds and flour)
- ✓ MILLET (high in protein, nice as hot cereal, used in soups, baking)
- ✓ LENTIL FLOUR (tasty, versatile, nutritious)
- ✓ QUINOA (very nutritious, delicious ancient grain)
- ✓ SORGHUM (wheat substitute in GF beer, baking flour)
- ✓ SOY (great in any form and as flour, high in protein)
- ✓ TAPIOCA FLOUR (used in pizza crusts, baking, from cassava root)
- ✓ TEFF (delicious ancient grain, flour, high in protein)
- ✓ YAM FLOUR (strong flavor)

# THE STRENGTHENING STUFF!
# (PROTEIN)

You don't need a lot of protein every day, but you do need some—about 10%-35%* of your daily intake. In fact, too much protein is stored as fat, so there is no need to binge on protein. Sources of protein include nuts, soybeans, beans, lentils, eggs, hard cheese and dairy, fish, whole grains and meat.

It is easy to prepare cooked meat. Once cooked thoroughly, it lasts up to three days covered in the fridge to use in other dishes and as a tasty sandwich using *Glee* bread.

When purchasing meat, check the expiration date. All meat must get in the freezer before that expiration date. Also, don't buy meat and then drive around for half an hour. You need to get it home to the fridge or freezer as soon as possible. *If it smells tangy, feels sticky/slimy, or starts to turn color*, toss it and wash your hands!

* USDA: National Agricultural Library. "Dietary Reference Intakes: Macronutrients." Food and Nutrition Information Center (2008).

Always wash your hands immediately after handling raw meat and wash everything (counter, knives, cutting boards) the raw meat touched.

To defrost frozen meat, follow microwave directions or leave in refrigerator 12–24 hours before cooking. Or you may leave frozen meat covered on a plate in a cool, dry spot out of direct sunlight until it is cold but no longer frozen.

> **WARNING:** Defrosting slowly at room temperature may expose meat to harmful bacteria.

## Chicken and Pork

Raw chicken and pork spoil easily. After you purchase the meat at the store, freeze it no matter what the expiration date says, unless you plan to use it (refrigerated) within 24 hours.

Both chicken and pork defrost pretty quickly (4–6 hours) with the exception of a whole chicken or pork roast which can take up to 24 hours to defrost in the fridge.

Cooked chicken or pork should be white in the middle, not pink. The dark meat on chicken (thighs) may appear brownish-pink in the middle, but should not be pink. To be on the safe side, purchase a meat thermometer at the grocery store and make sure the center temperature reaches 180°F.

If you prepare chicken or pork yourself, prepare enough for several different meals. Cooked chicken or pork will keep for up to three days in the fridge.

*To Prepare Grilled Chicken/Pork:*

---

It seems everyone has a George Foreman Grill in their dorm rooms and apartments these days. (Again, best to have your own, but if not, clean it before using.) For the *Glee* cook, I think it's a good idea to own a portable indoor grill, but follow the manufacturer's instructions.

The following instructions refer to an <u>outdoor gas grill</u>:

- To grill outdoors, use split chicken pieces (i.e., wings, thighs, breasts with bones) or boneless chicken pieces. Boneless pork chops and chops with bones are both fine.

- Scrape down grill rack.
- Lightly brush oil on the clean grill rack *and* on chicken or pork.
- Set grill 4"–5" above heat on MEDIUM and allow it to warm up for a few minutes.
- Place chicken or pork on grill rack over heat.
- Grill 12–15 minutes for a split chicken piece or pork chop <u>with</u> bones; or 5–7 minutes for <u>boneless</u> chicken or pork (clear juice should flow when you pierce it with a fork).
- Turn heat down to LOW and flip meat pieces over.
- Grill/broil another 10–12 minutes for chicken/pork <u>with bones</u>; 4–6 minutes for <u>boneless</u> chicken/pork.

**NOTE:** Try coating the chicken/pork with *Glee* marinade before grilling to prevent drying. Marinade recipes on page 156.

*To Prepare Broiled Chicken/Pork*

-----------------------------------------------------------------------

- Like grilled chicken/pork, use pieces with or without bones.

- Set oven rack at top (or next to top) level, 4"–5" below heat.

- Preheat broiler a minute or two.

- Place (lightly oiled) chicken/pork on broiler pan.

- Broil 12–15 minutes for a split chicken piece or pork chop <u>with</u> bones; or 5–7 minutes for <u>boneless</u> chicken or pork.

- Flip meat pieces over.

- Broil another 10–12 minutes for chicken/pork <u>with bones</u>; 4–6 minutes for <u>boneless</u> chicken/pork.

**NOTE:** Again, try coating the chicken/pork with *Glee* marinade before broiling to prevent drying. Marinade recipes on page 156.

*To Prepare Baked Chicken/Pork*

-----------------------------------------------------------------------

- Preheat oven to 350°F.

- Lightly oil a pan large enough for your chicken or pork pieces so that they barely touch each other.
- Lightly oil (salt & pepper) chicken or pork.
- Place pan of chicken or pork in the oven.
- Bake split chicken or pork chops (with bones) 45–55 minutes; 25–30 minutes for boneless pieces.
- Turn once halfway through baking.

**NOTE:** Again, tastes better with a marinade. See page 156.

*To Prepare Sautéed or Stir-Fried Chicken/Pork*

- Chop ½ lb boneless chicken or pork into bite-size pieces.
- Warm up 1 TBS oil in a frying pan or wok (tip pan/wok to coat with oil).
- Let pan/wok heat up on MED-HIGH.
- Toss in chicken or pork pieces and reduce heat to MEDIUM.
- Season with salt/pepper, garlic salt, ginger, and/or gluten-free soy sauce.

- Stir chicken or pork often until thoroughly cooked, 5–7 minutes.

*To Prepare Poach/Boiled (boneless chicken only)*

----------------------------------------------------------------

- Boil about 8–10 cups of water in a large pot.
- Once the water boils, throw in 1 TBS curry (optional), and about 4–6 boneless chicken pieces.
- The water will stop boiling, so wait until it begins boiling again.
- Turn pot down to MED-LOW and poach chicken pieces approx 12–15 minutes uncovered.
- Take chicken out of water and dry on paper towel (cut a piece in half and check to make sure center is white, not pink).
- Let cool for sandwiches or salads.

**NOTE:** Poached/Boiled pork is like rubber—I don't recommend it.

## To Prepare Roast Chicken

---

- Buy a whole chicken.

- Preheat oven to 350°F.

- Remove bag of giblets from the cavity and discard.

- Rinse the chicken thoroughly (inside and out) and dry with a paper towel.

- Place chicken in a roasting pan, breast side up.

- Stuff an apple or onion (cut in half) in the cavity of the chicken (discard after roasting).

- Tie the legs together with a bit of kitchen string, and then tie the wings.

- Spread pieces of butter or margarine all over the chicken skin, lightly salt and pepper.

- Slide prepared chicken into the preheated oven and ignore for the first hour.

- After one hour, baste the chicken every 20 minutes or so (i.e., spoon the juices from the pan over the top of the chicken a few times).

- Total roasting time is approximately 30 minutes/lb (ex: a 4 lb chicken will roast for approx 2 hours).

- (Optional: After the chicken has roasted for half the time—one hour for a 4 lb chicken—toss some par-boiled potatoes or carrots or turnip pieces around the chicken to roast.)

> **NOTE:** Many chickens come with a plastic thermometer which pops up out of the chicken when it is done. Or use a store-bought meat thermometer and cook chicken until the center meat temperature is 180°F.

*To Prepare Pork Roast*

- Preheat oven to 450°F.
- Rinse pork roast and pat dry.
- Place fat side up in lightly oiled roasting pan.
- Rub the outside with garlic and/or herbs (i.e., rosemary, sage or tarragon) and/or cover with thin layer of Dijon mustard.
- Reduce the oven temperature to 325°F.
- Cook pork roast approximately 30 minutes/lb (40 minutes/lb if it is rolled and tied or contains the bone).

- (Optional: Like a roast chicken, roast par-boiled potatoes or veggies in the pan with the pork.)

## Fish

---

Fish is wonderfully nutritious, low in calories and cholesterol–you've heard it all before! Try to eat fish in some form at least once a week. If you don't feel like cooking fish, eat canned tuna fish, sardines or salmon. If you despise fish, you may want to take high-quality fish oil capsules.

Below are basic instructions for plain, boneless fish fillets. Shellfish is also easy to cook–so look up a quick recipe.

*To Prepare Grilled/Broiled Fish*

------------------------------------------------------------

I prefer almost any fish on the grill. Fish also broils easily.

- Lightly oil the clean grill rack/broiler pan so the fillet doesn't stick.

**NOTE:** Many people prefer to grill/broil fish on lightly oiled aluminum foil as cooked fish burns and falls apart easily.

- Preheat grill/broiler a couple minutes.
- Fish fillets only need 3–5 minutes on each side at MEDIUM heat (longer for thicker fillets and fish steaks).
- Fish is done when cooked a uniform color and flakey inside when prodded with a fork.

*To Prepare Baked Fish*

- Preheat oven to 350°F.
- Place fish fillets in lightly greased glass dish or in pan on lightly greased aluminum foil.
- Bake 20–25 minutes (longer for thicker fillets and fish steaks) until fish flakes easily with a fork and is uniform in color.

**NOTE:** Experiment with marinades on fish or lightly coat in oil. Serve with toasted almonds for a delicious flavor.

## Beef

I once heard that salting beef (even hamburgers), then covering and placing the beef in the fridge for at least one hour and up to 12 hours, tenderizes it. And indeed it does! Just make sure you rinse the salt off before cooking the beef.

Hamburger can be scrambled in a pan and added to any dish, baked as a meatloaf (350°F for 45 minutes), and grilled or fried as burgers. You can cook the meat straight or add ketchup or egg or barbecue sauce to hamburger before cooking. Again, there are hundreds of recipes to look up.

Steaks (in a variety of cuts) are best grilled or broiled.

Stew meat is another versatile way to eat beef. You can stir-fry it in a pan (with a bit of oil to prevent sticking), slide it on shish-kabob and grill, or make a delicious easy stew in a slow cooker.

Beef is best cooked at a higher temperature in a shorter amount of time.

## To Prepare Beef Grilled Steak/Hamburger Patty

---

- Clean the grill.
- Preheat the grill a few minutes on HIGH.
- Grill steak for 6–10 minutes on MEDIUM depending on thickness (longer if there is a bone).
- Grill hamburger patty 5–6 minutes on MEDIUM.
- Flip and grill steak/patty same amount of time until desired level (rare/med/well).

## To Prepare Stir-fry

---

- Preheat pan (or wok) to a MED-HIGH temperature.
- Add 1 TBS oil (tip to coat pan/wok).

- Add and stir $^1/_2$ lb bite-size beef pieces until cooked, about 4–6 minutes.
- Remove and place on plate with paper towel to absorb oil.

**Instant/Quick Sources of Protein**

---

If you don't have time to prepare meat or prefer vegetarian options, the following foods provide instant sources of protein:

✓ Hummus (check ingredients)

✓ Peanut butter (also cashew, sunflower, and almond butters)

✓ Cheddar cheese

✓ Pre-cooked tofu (check ingredients)

✓ Yogurt

✓ Hard-boiled egg (already in your fridge)

✓ Handful of nuts/seeds

✓ Glass of milk (cow, goat, or soy)

✓ Cottage cheese

✓ Canned beans

✓ Canned chickpeas
✓ Lentil soup

## Easy Marinades for Grilling, Broiling, Baking

---

Chicken, pork, and fish are pretty dry and boring without marinades (or at least a little olive oil and salt/pepper) brushed on before cooking. Beef is usually tasty on its own, but marinades can also spice it up. There are hundreds of ideas in cookbooks and on the Internet, so experiment.

After cleaning and preparing raw chicken, pork, fish or beef, place in a deep bowl. Spread one of the suggested marinades (below) on both sides of your protein of choice before grilling, broiling or baking. Cover bowl, place in fridge from 15 minutes to 2 hours:

**C** = Chicken    **P** = Pork    **F** = Fish    **B** = Beef

- Annie's/Newman's Own (gluten-free) Barbecue Sauce **C/P/B**

- Annie's/Newman's Own (gluten-free) Salad Dressings (experiment with different ones) **C/P/F/B**
- $^1/_4$ cup olive oil mixed with 2 TBS red wine vinegar and 1 tsp lemon juice (experiment with adding herbs, such as basil or rosemary) **C/F**
- 1 cup whole yogurt mixed with 2 finely chopped garlic cloves (or 1 tsp dried garlic), 1 TBS lemon juice (experiment with adding herbs such as cumin, cilantro, dill or mint) **C/P/F**
- $^1/_2$ cup gluten-free soy sauce, $^1/_4$ cup gluten-free ketchup, $^1/_4$ cup brown sugar, 1 tsp powdered ginger **C/P**
- $^1/_4$ cup honey, 2 tsp gluten-free mustard, $^1/_4$ cup olive oil, 2 TBS lemon juice **C/P**
- Juice from 1 lime, 1 garlic clove minced, $^1/_2$ TBS olive oil **C/F**
- 3 TBS mustard, 1 TBS olive oil, minced garlic **C/P**

# THE COLORFUL STUFF!
## (VEGGIES, BEANS, AND FRUIT)

---

Vegetables/beans (legumes), and fruit should make up a substantial amount of your daily intake—in other words, you should consume approximately 2 $1/2$ cups of vegetables and 1 $1/2$ cups of fruit per day (including pure juices).* And listen, you need to eat vegetables even if you don't like them. If they make you gag, cut into tiny pieces, hide in your rice and add a bit of butter or shredded cheese. Eat them at least once a day, twice if possible.

### Frozen Vegetables

---

We always have packaged organic frozen vegetables in the freezer. They are already cut and ready to go, still loaded with vitamins and no additives. Boil/steam twice as much as you need and save the remainder in the fridge to add to other meals. (Follow easy directions on package.)

* For more information, visit www.mypyramid.gov.

## Fresh Vegetables

---

They are very nutritious raw, but some can be a bit hard on sensitive stomachs, especially the vegetable skins. You may find that you can't easily digest all fresh vegetables, such as carrots, but once steamed, boiled, baked, or stir-fried, they go down easier. Experiment with cooking them, adding diced or sliced vegetables anywhere. Poke with a fork to make sure they are desired tenderness.

**NOTE:** We always have fresh spinach in the fridge to eat raw as a salad or to add to cooking rice or in a pan when sautéing. Spinach is chock-full of those nutrients the *Glee* body needs, such as iron and folic acid with B-12.

## Salad

---

You must get in those dark greens everyday and it's easiest to do with a salad. If you find it annoying (as I do) to make a salad, chop up the whole head of lettuce and wash all the leaves at once in a spinner. Spin to dry and store in a container in the fridge; that way you can grab a handful whenever you want during the week. If bottled dressings generally bother your digestion, make a homemade dressing in a jar (see page 120). It will last several days.

## Beans/Legumes

So nutritious and easy to throw into any meal! Beans, a member of the *Legume* family, are easy to cook (follow simple directions on bag/box) or purchase canned. They are high in protein, fiber, iron and minerals, and low in fat, calories, and contain no cholesterol. Some of the more common beans are the black, kidney, lima, and navy varieties. Lentils, peanuts, soy nuts, chickpeas, and peas, also members of the *Legume* family, contain similar nutritional benefits.

## Fruit

Almost everyone likes at least two or three kinds of fruit. Always choose fresh fruit over canned fruit or fruit juice. If you drink juice, go for pure juice with pulp, not concentrate.

Again, some of you *Glee* eaters may have a tough time with the skin of fruit, like peaches and pears, so you may need to peel them. If you do eat the skins you should always eat organic. Fruit with thinner exteriors, such as grapes and strawberries, should always be organic (due to invasive pesticides).

If a particular fruit bothers you, such as apples, you may find it easier to digest it cooked (like applesauce) or baked in a *Glee* muffin or bread.

## Dried Fruit

Almost every fruit can be purchased dried (i.e., all the water has been removed) in a package or sold in bulk in a bin. These tasty morsels are packed with nutrients. Brigitte particularly likes dried apricots. They make a quick snack or nice addition to rice dishes and salads. In addition to the good, old raisin, other popular dried fruits are tomatoes, bananas, cranberries, figs, dates, and cherries.

# Instant/Quick Source of Veggies, Beans, and Fruit

If you don't have time to cook or make a salad, the following foods provide an instant or quick source of vegetable, beans, or fruit:

✓ Raw vegetables

✓ Raw fruit

✓ Pure vegetable or tomato juice

✓ Pure fruit juice (with pulp)

✓ Dried fruit

✓ Tomato sauce (over prepared GF pasta or brown rice)

✓ Frozen vegetables

✓ Vegetable GF soup

✓ Canned beans

✓ Peanut butter

✓ Bean GF soup

✓ Lentil GF soup

✓ Fresh GF salsa

# A FRIENDLY REMINDER...

Whether you have celiac disease or you are giving up gluten for other medical reasons, this reference guide offers no promises, only suggestions. It is up to you to verify the ingredients of everything that goes into your mouth. To summarize there are several ways to do this:

- Contact a reputable celiac disease association.
- Join a CD product newsletter.
- Subscribe online to a regularly updated gluten-free product list.
- Search well-established gluten-free websites.
- Search websites of food manufacturers—many include gluten-free information.
- Pick up the phone and call the toll-free number printed on any package.

Most packaged foods, medicines and products are not manufactured on a dedicated gluten-free line or in a dedicated gluten-free facility. In the end, it is you who must make the final gastronomical decision.

*Wonderful Websites*

# ONLINE *GLEE* FOOD SUPPLIERS

- www.againstthegraingourmet.com (absolutely delicious bagels/breads)
- www.amazon.com (lots of GF foods)
- www.amyskitchen.com (terrific microwavable/toaster oven meals)
- www.bionaturae.com (organic pastas from Italy)
- www.bobsredmill.com (variety of GF whole grain products)
- www.chebe.com (specialized GF bread products and mixes)
- www.ener-g.com (huge variety)
- www.enjoylifefoods.com (our favorite cookies, breakfast bars)
- www.envirokidz.com (breakfast cereal)
- www.fantasticfoods.com (ready-made GF food)
- www.foodsbygeorge.com (pizza and brownies)
- www.freedavitamins.com (GF vitamins)
- www.gfgreatbakes.com (known for their bagels)
- www.glutenfree.com (all sorts of baked goods and breads/crackers)

- www.glutenfreebagelcompany.com (great bagels)
- www.glutenfreemall.com (ships practically everything *Glee*)
- www.glutino.com (baked goods, pizzas and more)
- www.naturemade.com (GF vitamins)
- www.reallygreatfoods.com (bread machine and bakery mixes)
- www.traderjoes.com (online gluten-free list)
- www.vansintl.com (waffles)
- www.wegmans.com (online GF product list)
- www.wholefoodsmarket.com (gluten-free "Bake House")

# MAINSTREAM FOOD COMPANIES

The following are short lists of HUGE and not-so-huge food and household manufacturers who make and sell some of your favorite condiments, packaged foods, household and ready-to-eat products.

Some of the companies listed below provide gluten-free information on their websites. You may have to click on specific product websites for gluten-free information or you may need to call the consumer line.

> **WARNING:** Most of the "food and household products" manufactured by the following companies are NOT produced in gluten-free dedicated facilities.

## The Biggies

- KRAFT: www.kraftfoods.com
- HEINZ: www.heinz.com
- HORMEL: www.hormel.com

- FRITO-LAY: www.fritolay.com
- NESTLE: www.nestleusa.com
- PROCTOR & GAMBLE: www.pg.com
- SARA LEE: www.saralee.com

## Smaller Companies

---

Check the following websites for gluten-free information or call the company directly:

- ANNIE'S: www.annies.com
- BARBARA'S BAKERY: www.worldpantry.com
- IAN'S NATURAL FOODS: www.iansnaturalfoods.com
- LUNDBERG FAMILY FARMS: www.lundberg.com
- MAPLE GROVE FARMS: www.maplegrove.com
- NATURE'S PATH: www.naturespath.com
- NEWMAN'S OWN: www.newmansown.com
- WOLFGANG PUCK: www.wolfgangpuck.com

# ADDITIONAL *GLEE* WEBSITES

## Non-Profit Organizations

- ⌖ www.americanceliac.org
- ⌖ www.csaceliacs.org
- ⌖ www.celiac.org
- ⌖ www.celiaccentral.org
- ⌖ www.gluten.net
- ⌖ www.healthyvilli.org

## Magazines/Newsletters

- ⌖ Gluten-Free Living: www.glutenfreeliving.com
- ⌖ Living Without: www.livingwithout.com
- ⌖ Online Magazine: www.glutenfreeda.com
- ⌖ Online Newsletter: www.clanthompson.com
- ⌖ Online Newsletter: www.celiac.com ("Scott-Free")

**NOTE:** Almost all celiac disease foundations have some type of publication.

## GF Product Lists

---

- 🖱 www.csaceliacs.org
- 🖱 www.clanthompson.com
- 🖱 www.celiac.com

## Traveling/Dining Out

---

- 🖱 www.aoecs.org (Association of European Coeliac Societies)
- 🖱 www.bobandruths.com (dining and travel club)
- 🖱 www.celiachandbook.com (excellent restaurant source)
- 🖱 www.clanthompson.com (mini pocket guides available to purchase)
- 🖱 www.clanthompson.com (click on "Lifestyle", then "Travel")
- 🖱 www.gluten-free-onthego.com
- 🖱 www.glutenfreemeals.com (meals delivered to your door)
- 🖱 www.glutenfreepassport.com (book series)

- <sup>🖱</sup> www.glutenfreeregistry.com (national list of restaurants, bakeries, etc)
- <sup>🖱</sup> www.glutenfreerestaurants.org
- <sup>🖱</sup> www.celiactravel.com (includes restaurant card in many languages)

## College-Bound

---

- <sup>🖱</sup> www.celiacdisease.net (includes honor roll of gluten-free friendly colleges)
- • Celiac Info Line at University of Chicago Celiac Disease Center: (773)702-7593

## Medical Contacts

---

- <sup>🖱</sup> Boston Celiac Center at Beth Israel Deaconess Medical Center: www.bidmc.harvard.edu
- <sup>🖱</sup> Celiac Disease Center at Columbia University: www.celiacdiseasecenter.columbia.edu
- <sup>🖱</sup> University of Chicago Celiac Disease Program: www.uchospitals.edu

🖱 University of Maryland Center of Celiac Research: www.celiaccenter.org

**Don't Forget...**

---

Please donate to the non-profit online *Glee* organizations mentioned on these pages whenever possible—or at the very least, e-mail them a quick thank-you! They have done heaps of research and provide such a valuable service.

# BIBLIOGRAPHY

## Internet Sources

www.abilitymagazine.com/celiac–general

www.americanceliac.org–resources, advocacy, labeling

www.celiac.com–candy, general, R.O.C.K. (Raising Our
   Celiac Kids), general

www.celiac.org–general

www.celiaccentral.org–general, candy

www.celiactravel.com–travel, food cards

www.uchospitals.edu/specialties/celiac–medical
   information

www.clanthompson.com–over-the-counter drug list,
   candy list, food lists

www.csaceliacs.org–CSA Gluten-Free Product Listing
   Manual, general

www.fda.gov–US Food Labeling Laws

www.gfcfdiet.com–toothpaste, cosmetics, cleaners,
   condiments

www.glutenfreeandeasy.com–GF foods

www.glutenfreeclub.com–sodas

www.glutenfreedrugs.com–over-the-counter drug list

www.keepkidshealthy.com–general, Italy

www.mayoclinic.com/health/legumes–beans

www.mypyramid.gov–nutritional info

www.npr.org–"For Most People, Gluten Isn't a Diet Enemy" (5/10/07)

www.pechsiam.com/allabout.htm–rice info

www.usda.gov–nutritional requirements

www.wellness.gatech.edu–protein

www.wholegrainscouncil.org–rice/grains

## Books

---

Adamson, Eve and Tricia Thompson. The Complete Idiot's Guide to Gluten-Free Eating. New York: Alpha Books, 2007.

Bower, Sylvia Llewelyn. A Guide to Living with Gluten Intolerance. New York: Demos Medical Publishing, 2007.

Case, Shelley. Gluten-Free Diet. Saskatchewan, Canada: Case Nutrition Consulting, 2006.

Green, Peter H.R. Celiac Disease: A Hidden Epidemic.
New York: HarperCollins, 2006.

Korn, Danna. Living Gluten-Free for Dummies.
Indianapolis, IN: Wiley Publishing, Inc, 2006.

Lieberman, Shari. The Gluten Connection. New York:
Rodale, Inc, 2007.

London, Melissa. The GF Kid: A Celiac Disease
Survival Guide. Bethesda, MD: Woodbine House,
2005.

Lowell, Jax Peters. The Gluten-Free Bible. New York:
Henry Holt & Co, 2005.

Maltin, Vanessa. Beyond Rice Cakes. Bloomington, IN:
IUniverse, 2006.

Neena and Veena, The Way of the Belly. Carlsbad, CA:
Hay House, 2006.

Thompson, Tricia. Gluten-Free Nutrition Guide. New
York: McGraw-Hill, 2008.

## Other

---

Clan Thomson Food SmartList 2009.

Ratner, Amy. "Colleges Take on the Gluten-Free Diet."
Gluten-Free Living Magazine. Vol 11: No. 2, 2007.

Thompson, Lani K. Celiac Pocket Guide: Food,
Restaurants, Over the Counter Drugs, Prescription
Drugs, Beer, Wine & Spirits, Everything Else. Bridg-
ton, ME: Clan Thompson Publisher, 2007.

Whelan, Ann, ed. "Gluten-Free Living Magazine".
Hawthorne, NY: Jan–Dec 2007.

# ACKNOWLEDGEMENTS

Simplifying a topic like celiac disease takes a heap of work with help from many people. I would like to thank Jocelyne Cosentino for being the first to gently educate our family about CD and for reading _Glee!_ with special attention to the food combos and recipes. Jennifer Leonard-Solis, an editor and writer extraordinaire, provided a layman's analytical eye. Susan Cohen lent her literary and marketing expertise, while Lauren Komack (board member of the Healthy Villi) closely reviewed the manuscript. My mom, Bobbi Atkinson, passed on her nutritional common sense with lots of love, as well as proofed the basic recipes. A special thanks to Lani and Jeff Thompson for taking on this project and for providing such a valuable service to thousands of people. And as always, thanks to my patient husband, Erik Eames, for giving me the writer's life . . . and of course my old black lab, China, for keeping me company.

# MY *GLEE* NOTES

# ABOUT THE AUTHOR

**Elizabeth Atkinson**, author of the tween novel *From Alice to Zen and Everyone in Between*, researched celiac disease with a passion when her daughter was diagnosed in 2006. When she realized there was a need for an easy survival guide for young adults and newly diagnosed adults, she immediately set to work creating a concise and upbeat book. The author divides her time between West Newbury, Massachusetts and Center Lovell, Maine. For more information visit her website at www.elizabethatkinson.com.

# ABOUT THE PUBLISHER

**Clan Thompson** is a family business owned and operated by Lani and Jeff Thompson. When Lani's husband, Dave, was first diagnosed with celiac disease around 1994, she began researching which foods were safe for him to eat. Soon Jeff was also diagnosed and eventually seven Thompsons were found to have celiac disease! There wasn't much information available back then, and the Thompson clan soon realized that the information they were collecting would be useful to other celiacs as well. Their pocket guides and SmartList software covers verified gluten information on more than 20,000 products. For more information, visit their website at www.clanthompson.com.

Breinigsville, PA USA
01 October 2009
225118BV00004B/3/P